# The suffering gene

## About the author

**Roy Burdon** has been Emeritus Professor at the University of Strath-clyde since 1997, where he was previously Chairman of the Department of Bioscience and Biotechnology. He served as a member of the editorial boards of several journals, such as *The Biochemical Journal*, *Nucleic Acids Research*, *The Scottish Medical Journal*, *Free Radicals in Biology and Medicine* and *The Biological Sciences Review*. He is an author of more than two hundred scientific papers, and also of a number of books, including *RNA Biosynthesis* (1976, Chapman & Hall), *The Molecular Biology of DNA Methylation* (1989, Springer Verlag) and *Genes and the Environment* (1999, Taylor & Francis). He was Chairman of the Biochemical Society and is a Fellow of the Royal Society of Edinburgh.

# The suffering gene

## Environmental threats
## to our health

**ROY BURDON**

McGILL–QUEEN'S UNIVERSITY PRESS
*Montreal and Kingston · London · Ithaca*

DAVID PHILIP
*Cape Town*

ZED BOOKS
*London & New York*

*The Suffering Gene* was first published by
Zed Books Ltd, 7 Cynthia Street, London N1 9JF, UK,
and Room 400, 175 Fifth Avenue, New York, NY 10010, USA, in 2003
www.zedbooks.demon.co.uk

Published in South Africa by David Philip (Pty Ltd),
99 Garfield Road, Claremont 7700

Published in Canada by McGill-Queen's University Press,
3430 McTavish Street, Montreal, QC H3A 1X9

Cover designed by Andrew Corbett
Designed and typeset in Monotype Garamond by Illuminati, Grosmont, UK
Printed and bound in the EU by Gutenberg Printers Ltd, Malta

Distributed in the USA exclusively by Palgrave, a division of
St Martin's Press, LLC, 175 Fifth Avenue, New York, NY 10010

A catalogue record for this book is available from the British Library

US CIP data is available from the Library of Congress

National Library of Canada Cataloguing in Publication Data
Burdon, R.H. (Roy Hunter)
    The suffering gene : environmental threats to our health / Roy Burdon.
    Includes bibliographical references and index.
    ISBN 0–7735–2655–2 (bound).—ISBN 0–7735–2656–0 (pbk.)
    1. Cancer—Etiology.  2. Genetic toxicology.  3. Carcinogens.  4. Environmental
toxicology.  5. Cancer—Environmental aspects.  6. Environmentally induced
diseases.  I. Title.
    RA1224.3.B87 2003          616.99'4071          C2003-901624-2

In South Africa
ISBN 0 86486 627 5 Pb

In Canada
ISBN 0 7735 2655 2 Hb
ISBN 0 7735 2656 0 Pb

In the Rest of the World
ISBN 1 84277 284 8 Hb
ISBN 1 84277 285 6 Pb

# Contents

# Figures and tables

# Acknowledgements

I have benefited significantly, over many years, from the experience and expertise of a host of professional scientific colleagues and personal friends. For their advice and wisdom I shall always be grateful. A crucial comment from some was that it would be valuable if a short book could be written, readily accessible to the layperson, which explained the ways in which our genes are now besieged by an array of environmental adversities. To this end, in *The Suffering Gene* I have endeavoured to explain simply what genes are, how they work, and the consequences for them and us in the face of such environmental threats. In the book's preparation, I have to acknowledge the patience, help and unstinting encouragement from Robert Molteno and the editorial staff at Zed Books, together with the unfailing patience and support of my wife, Margery, who made proofreading and other essential corrections as painless as possible.

# Early warning signals

The days grow longer and warmer as spring follows winter. Each year, buds appear on the trees, leaves and flowers form, and seeds develop; life and growth surge up in plants and animals. We are part of a system that seems to behaves like a machine, constantly repeating itself, season by season, year by year. Yet, as we enter a new millennium, there are signs that the workings of this machine cannot be taken for granted. The environment is certainly at present not in anything approaching meltdown, but all is not well. Few days go past without media reports on climate change, ozone depletion, chemical and oil spills, radiation leaks, massive deforestation and deleterious changes in land use. Plant and animal species are becoming extinct at a rate that is much more rapid than at any previous time. Estimates of losses are hotly debated, varying between as many as 4,000 and 14,000 species each year. Many of these alarming events have been triggered by human efforts to modify the natural environment to create new land for agriculture, industry and dwellings. We are now very dependent on the diversity of plant, animal and microbial species for a whole range of essential services, including the recycling of atmospheric gases, water and nutrients, as well as clothing, shelter and medicines. It is only just over thirty years ago that photographs from the Apollo missions to the moon gave the very first glimpse of planet Earth in its entirety. These images were appealingly serene and inspirational, but the real picture differs and offers little comfort. Human activity has recently set in motion changes capable of fundamentally altering our planet's natural systems in unprecedented ways. Global change is very much on the menu.

Although most of us live in cities, somewhat removed from farms and the countryside, our heavy dependence on plants is evident from our enormous use of fabrics, paper, timber, medicines and, particularly, food. The acquisition of the knowledge that enabled man to live in this way began when our early ancestors learned to distinguish edible plants from poisonous ones and started to create useful things from wood and other plant products. *Homo sapiens* reached the western hemisphere around 30,000 BC and was presented with possible new types of food plants and immense herds of game. During this period, he was simply a part of the natural relationship between hunters and the hunted. Mankind had serious enemies, such as sabre-toothed tigers. However, by about 8,000 BC man stood on the brink of the transition from a hunter–gatherer society to one based on agriculture. Evidence suggests that this took place in the so-called 'Fertile Crescent' located in the hills between Israel, Jordan, Turkey, Syria, Iran and Iraq, the home of wild barley and wild wheat. Groups of hunters may have cleared areas around their camps to gain protection from enemies or predators. New plants would have sprung up in such clearings. Some of these would be of direct use to the encamped families, while others would attract game, beginning the process of animal husbandry. At that time, the animals most responsive to domestication were dogs (for hunting), goats, sheep, cattle, pigs and horses (for meat and hide). Over most of Europe, at least, the transition from hunting to farming appears to have been very rapid. Once the initial steps had been taken, agriculture allowed the population to increase dramatically. By 8,000 BC, it had taken *Homo sapiens* 90,000 years to reach a global population of around 5 million. In the next 1,500 years this figure doubled. By 1850 it was 1,300 million. A further 400 million was added to this figure in the next fifty years. Between 1930 and 1975 the world's population again doubled to around 3,900 million. If the growth rate of the last few decades (1.9 per cent) continues unabated, then there will be over 7,000 million people by the year 2010.

We have taken our planet very much for granted throughout most of our history. However, in the nineteenth century Victorian society developed a grand passion for natural history – the study of nature. This sometimes manifested itself in bizarre excesses such as butterfly mania, aquarium fever and gorilla madness. Those with social aspirations ventured into the countryside in grand parties, or invited their fashionable friends around for 'an evening at the microscope'. Some felt their drawing rooms to be incomplete without strange stuffed birds, unusual insect collections or exotic ferns. This study of nature was believed to lead to spiritual enlightenment. Myriads of plant and animal species were avidly collected and catalogued. Fossils were hunted out in large numbers at a time when our understanding of the earth's geology was beginning to blossom. Together these activities served to create a solid and intellectually enlightened society that laid the foundations of our present-day understanding of evolution and ecology. *Evolution* describes the processes that have transformed life on our planet from its earliest forms to the enormous diversity of today. *Ecology* relates the interactions between organisms and their environment. In the next century, thanks to those timely studies of our Victorian forebears, it gradually became clear that human activities could have undesirable effects on the complex and delicate relationships that exist between living organisms and their habitats.

For the foreseeable future, earth is our only place of abode. Moreover, we share it with a vast diversity of other living organisms. We are unique; only we can appreciate the predicament that faces the planet and thus responsibility for its future well-being rests firmly on our shoulders. From earliest times the environment has impacted on our daily activities. Agricultural success was achieved despite often adverse climatic conditions. Floods and droughts as well as the ravages of insects and other predators all took their toll on productivity. Nowadays the growth of urbanized societies has led to the industrialization of agriculture. This is highly dependent on the use of pesticides and fertilizers at high levels for intensive cultivation, together with the extensive use of pharmaceutical products in livestock husbandry. Over the past two hundred years or so we have brought about fundamental changes to the chemical environment. In the middle of the eighteenth century, steam power became the dominant energy source of industrial civilization. Carbon-based fuels such as coal, peat, oil, and natural gas are burned in large quantities, releasing complex chemical mixtures into the air, water and soils. These fuels are also used by the petrochemical and manufacturing industry to produce the raw materials for synthetic consumer products such as plastics, paint, dyes, pharmaceuticals, cosmetics, food and food additives. Not only does each process release waste chemicals into the environment; once used, the products themselves are excreted, dumped or burned, further contributing to the overall load of synthetic chemicals in the environment.

## Going to work can be dangerous

As consumers we seem to have become hopelessly addicted to the comforts of our industrialized modern lifestyle. However, the costs of our regular 'fixes' are rising and there is no 'detox' therapy readily available. The writing has been on the wall for some time. For many centuries it has been known that exposure to some substances in the workplace can have adverse effects on the health of people working with them. Early civilizations responded to this not by making the work any safer, but by using it as a punishment for slaves and criminals, or relegating the work to the lowest classes of their people. In Roman times, forced labour in the Spanish cinnabar mines was regarded as the equivalent to a death sentence. This was due to exposure of the luckless prisoners to mercury. In *Alice's Adventures in Wonderland* by Lewis Carroll, the Mad Hatter demonstrated many of the neurological symptoms associated with mercury poisoning. This probably arose from the treatment of rabbit fur with mercury to create the felt used in the manufacture of hats. The expression 'as mad as a hatter' can be traced to the mental condition of some workers in this industry.

## All substances can be viewed as poisons

By the fifteenth and sixteenth centuries, it was known that mine workers suffered a variety of diseases as a direct consequence of their employment. This was thought to be due to the dusts, stagnant air and the gases found in the mines. Today we recognize these diseases as pneumoconiosis, tuberculosis and lung cancer. In 1567 a physician with the grand name Phillippus Aureolus Theophrastus Bombastus von Hohenheim-Paracelsus established the crucial concept that all substances are poisons. There is none which is not a poison. The right dose differentiates a poison and a remedy. Paracelsus can be viewed as the founding father of modern toxicology and was responsible for establishing the concept of a 'dose–response' relationship. In his view it was essential to evaluate our responses to chemicals and to make a distinction between beneficial and toxic properties of substances. The fact that all substances are potential poisons is a theme to which we will return later. For the moment some examples will suffice. To alleviate the symptoms of a wide variety of ailments many of us take small doses of aspirin with hardly a thought. Yet we know that large doses of the same substance can be fatal. Coffee can be a marvellous pick-me-up, but excessive coffee drinking can have unwanted effects on behaviour and sleep patterns. Kitchen salt as a flavour enhancer at mealtimes is fine in small doses, but if taken to excess can have undesirable effects on blood pressure.

## Workplace medicine

By the beginning of the eighteenth century, diseases of the workplace were increasingly becoming a matter of concern. With the publication of Bernadino Ramazzini's dissertation on Diseases of Occupation   (*De Morbis Artificium Diatriba*), occupational medicine effectively became an independently recognized discipline. Ramazzini (1633–1714) systematically examined a number of occupations and trades, paying particular attention to the prevailing conditions of work and the diseases suffered in these situations. Because of this study, he was able to suggest a number of changes to working practices that concerned workers' welfare: hygiene, posture, ventilation and protective clothing. Many of his recommendations are as valid today as they were in the early 1700s. He urged that doctors, when taking a patient's history, should remember the key question, 'What is you occupation?' The answer could often contribute enormously to the successful diagnosis of the patient's condition.

In 1775, the British physician Percival Pott noted a curious prevalence of ragged sores on the scrotums of many chimney sweeps then at work in London. Other doctors could easily have dismissed the matter, assuming that the men were simply afflicted with venereal disease, then rampant throughout the city. Pott was more astute, realizing that they were in fact suffering from a type of skin cancer.

This discovery was a major medical milestone. By observing that men continually exposed to the chemicals in soot were 'peculiarly liable' to this form of cancer, he was able to document for the first time that human cancer could be caused by environmental agents. It is now well known that soot owes its cancer-causing properties to tar, and that one of the principal culprits is a substance called *benzpyrene*. As we shall see later, this chemical has the ability to enter cells and tissues and cause modifications to the DNA of our genes, initiating the chain of events that ultimately leads to the development of cancers.

Despite such enlightenment, conditions did not improve rapidly in the workplace. Between 1760 and 1830, Britain embraced the Industrial Revolution wholeheartedly. Workers no longer owned the means of production; the demand for goods had grown to such an extent that mass production was the only answer. Mainly this was achieved through the use of machines such as the 'Spinning Jenny' of James Hargreave, which could do the work of many individual workers. These machines had to be housed in large mills and factories. In turn these generated an increase in the use of chemicals such as acids, alkalis, soaps and mordants necessary for the processing of textiles. In short, conditions were created for vastly increased exposure of workers to hazardous substances.

Despite the radical changes in working practices that characterized the Industrial Revolution, there were still physicians in the UK dedicated to occupational hygiene. For example Charles Thackray (1795–1831) was concerned with the diseases among the working classes of Leeds, and he was able to recommend the elimination of lead used as a glaze in the pottery industry, as well as the use of ventilation and respiratory protection for knife grinders. In fact, he was probably the first physician in the English-speaking world to practise occupational medicine. Through his many writings, he was able to publicize his findings widely and thus the general public became more aware of the wretched conditions of the working classes. Circumstances in the factories and mills at that time were often appalling. Thanks to the efforts of enlightened and highly qualified crusaders like Charles Thackray and fellow Victorians, the Factory Act of 1833 and the Mines Act of 1842 eventually passed through parliament.

Notwithstanding these great legislative advances, conditions in the workplace still continued to be highly hazardous. By the second half of the nineteenth century, new industries were coming on-stream that brought with them a new set of dangers. Cutlers and potters were dying prematurely of diseases brought on by silicon-based substances. In the manufacture of Lucifer matches, workers were exposed to white phosphorus, which caused necrosis of the jaw. The general public was also not entirely safe. Newspapers of the day carried reports that the new aniline dyes, which were very much a growth industry, could cause skin inflammations. Some of these novel dyes were used for cloths and wallpapers, and scares abounded regarding the safety of dyed ball gowns and stockings. Although some dyestuffs, as will be mentioned later in this book, were subsequently found to be hazardous for other reasons, the problem of the skin inflammations was traced to small amounts of arsenic that remained in the dyes. During dye manufacture, arsenic was sometimes used, but occasionally it was not completely filtered off and washed away. A minute contamination of arsenic could nonetheless be problematic in damp conditions, especially if the wearer of the dyed clothes was prone to perspiration.

Despite such clear warning signals, human activity over the last hundred years has accelerated the creation of an increasingly diverse and malevolent chemical environment. Unfortunately there is growing evidence of a veritable cocktail of potentially hostile environmental chemicals in the air, as well as in water and food.

## An unscheduled experiment

At the same time as Dr Pott was studying scrotal cancer in chimney sweeps, Georgian England had a legal system that inflicted severe punishments for petty crimes: forgery or thievery often resulted in a death sentence, a ludicrously harsh punishment. A backlash against such a sentence for what were relatively trivial misdemeanours led to milder punishments, but the jails were soon filled to capacity. To thin out what was really an underclass of small-time thieves and to unburden the country's prisons, the House of Commons voted at the beginning of the 1780s to banish its less desirable citizens to some remote locale. They chose Australia, at that time a little-known shore bordering the South Pacific Ocean, first visited by the then Lieutenant James Cook in 1770.

Remarkably, the British parliament's decision to transport large batches of petty criminals was taken without any further reconnoitering of the Australian coast. The First Fleet, as it became known, nonetheless set off from Portsmouth in 1787, comprising eleven ships and a complement of around 1,500, which included 700 prisoners, together with the ships' crew and officers, officers' families, as well as the governor and his staff. For most of the prisoners the period of exile was set at seven years, but, since few had any possibility of raising the return fare, banishment to Australia was effectively a life sentence.

Within a few decades the east coast of Australia was heavily populated with British and Irish men and women. These early colonists often shared the Celtic features of fair skin and light hair, and today their descendants predominate on that southern continent. What began as an eighteenth-century attempt at penal reform ultimately culminated in a large-scale, but unscheduled, experiment specifically linking sunlight and skin cancer.

It is now well understood that exposure to the radiation from the sun can cause severe damage to eyes and skin. The lenses of our eyes are prone to accumulating damage caused by sunlight and, although initially transparent, can become cloudy, forming a cataract. Skin can be readily burned and inflamed following exposure to excessive sunlight. It can lose its elasticity and become wrinkled as if prematurely aged, and, in extreme conditions, become deeply furrowed and lumpy. More serious is the possibility of developing skin cancers after prolonged exposure. Many of these cancers are fatal. They result from the damage caused by the ultraviolet component of solar radiation to certain genes within skin cells that normally control orderly growth, so that they are permitted to multiply out of control and spread widely throughout the body. In the last forty years there has been a worrying increase in a particularly aggressive type of skin cancer (malignant melanoma) in the white populations of countries such as Britain, the USA and Australia. With their fair skin continually exposed to intense sun, whites in Australia now have the highest rates of all kinds of skin cancer of any people in the world. Their British relatives, who live under cloudy northern skies, have a lower risk of acquiring these cancers.

## About this book

Many other environmental hazards, besides sunlight, are causing increasing concern because of their ability to damage genes and cause cancers (Table 1.1). As well as the possibility of initiating cancers, damage to genes can have other long-term consequences. A faulty gene can be inherited by future generations. Offspring can become more susceptible to cancers, or be burdened with genetic diseases that prejudice their ability to cope with life, or, indeed, their survival. A crucial question is whether we will be able to adapt to these and other environmental changes, or whether we will pay a severe price in terms of declining health and the uncertain survival of future generations.

Our interactions with the environment are complex, but crucial aspects are the many ways in which environmental components can attack genes, which can have significant consequences for health and welfare both in the short and the long term.

This book aims to explain the nature of genes and why we should be concerned for their well-being. Genes are under continual attack, not only from a range of environmental adversities but also from processes going on within our own bodies. Fortunately we have many

**Table 1.1**   Environmental hazards that can damage genes

| | |
|---|---|
| Sunlight | From ultraviolet radiation |
| Nuclear radiation | From nuclear power stations, reprocessing plants, X-rays, rocks and soil |
| Atmospheric pollutants | Combustion of fossil fuels such as coal, oil, petrol |
| | Tobacco smoke |
| | Automobile exhaust |
| | Asbestos |
| | Ozone |
| Food components | Contaminants from fungi |
| | Cooking products |
| Synthetic chemicals | Various industrial products (e.g. aluminium, iron, steel and coke; dyestuffs, rubber, pesticides, paints, plastics, pharmaceuticals, cosmetics, food additives) |
| Therapeutic drugs | Anticancer agents |

ways of defending genes from such attacks. We can also make 'running repairs' to genes that suffer damage, and although the effectiveness of such protection and repair can vary considerably between individuals, additional protection can nonetheless be bought in the shape of components of our daily diet.

The question of how best to survive this siege on our genes is addressed in the chapters that follow, as is the risk of developing various types of cancer that can sometimes result if our defences are breached. The pressing need for a more rigorous evaluation and awareness of the increasing hazards of synthetic chemicals in the environment is emphasized. The question of whether the ongoing siege suffered by genes might somehow redirect the future evolution of the human species is also examined. Certainly the possibility that the environment might influence evolution did exercise the minds of a considerable number of eminent biologists in the nineteenth and twentieth centuries. Although it is now accepted that the environment cannot *specifically* direct evolution, it is clear that the action, as well as the structure, of many genes can be profoundly influenced by environmental factors. Altered genes are nonetheless crucial to evolution. They serve as the basis of the genetic variation among populations of organisms that is necessary for the evolutionary processes of natural selection to proceed. However, as we shall see, these processes are not specifically directed. Moreover, they operate over a timescale, which is almost infinitely long in comparison to the short time that encompasses the sorts of environmental adversity described in this book. Fears for our long-term evolutionary future from environmental challenges are probably unfounded, in the present circumstances. More likely is the possibility of more immediate health problems such as cancers and other debilitating, sometimes hereditary, conditions.

Although we may be rightly concerned with the ongoing environmental siege directed at our own genes, this could be seen as purely self-centred. We have been engaged in 'robbing' other species of their genes for some time now. Over many thousands of years, this assault on the genes of other species has been part of our history and culture, and has been carried out in the name of agricultural improvement. Effectively we have been stealing genes from a variety of wild plants and animals and transferring them to other organisms, in the normal course of breeding more productive domestic agricultural stock. However, in the last twenty-five years we have been able to develop technologies that will allow us to refine this approach enormously. Previous breeding strategies had to rely on the random nature of genetic assortment that was part of the normal fertilization processes involving eggs and sperm. With the advent of genetic engineering, it is now possible to short-circuit this time-consuming and unpredictable process. In the laboratory we can snip out the requisite gene from one species and insert it directly into another. It is now possible for us to create combinations of genes never before seen in nature. In so doing, we can effectively lay siege to millions of years of evolutionary history. Put another way, the particular genes and their arrangements that characterize individual species and that are the culmination of the intricate and enormously lengthy processes of evolution can now be raided in a matter of hours. New gene arrangements can be quickly created that cut across previously established evolutionary barriers.

This new technology of genetic engineering has nonetheless raised the hope of using genes as medicines in the treatment of inherited human diseases. The possibility of cutting out the defective gene from a disease victim and replacing it with its normal equivalent has stimulated much public interest. For a variety of reasons, this possibility has not yet materialized, but the techniques, together with recent developments in cloning, have raised the possibility of what the popular press calls 'designer babies'. The concept of a 100 per cent healthy baby of the preferred gender and with the desired genetic composition has a particular fascination for the human mind as far as can be judged from the pages of science fiction. Whilst there are many practical, political and ethical barriers, the possibility of genetically engineering offspring more able to tolerate environmental stress has its attractions. Although the present environmental adversities may seem bearable, there is always the possibility of a more serious decline in our planetary conditions. This is not mere speculation. Already the world has faced five episodes of mass extinction during which environmental extremes forced the demise of many plant and animal species. According to some, a sixth period of extinction may already be under way and our long-term survival may be in jeopardy. Trawling the genetic resources of many animals, plants and microbes sharing our planet has thrown up an impressive catalogue of genes that play key roles in resisting a variety of very significant environmental stresses. Some of these so-called stress genes could conceivably form the basis of an escape package if environmental conditions became seriously life threatening and a quick fix were required. Although our present technical skills are wholly inadequate, it might be possible at some time in the future to engineer stress-tolerant offspring incorporating the most effective of these genes.

All these ideas could properly be dismissed as wishful, or woolly, thinking, the stuff of science fiction. Certainly the evaluation of their potential usefulness can only follow a proper appreciation of our present predicament. Governments and health authorities do attach a growing importance to an accurate understanding of the increasing threats arising from the environment. A consideration of these from the perspective of our genes is especially timely. There has been extensive international research collaboration that has just recently been able to reveal details of all our genes and how they are arranged. This can be looked upon as the basic set of instructions, or recipe, that governs the way we are constructed, and how we function. It has been referred to by some as the Book of Life and is likely to yield far-reaching insights into the basis of disease as well as telling us much about our origins and history on planet earth.

Increasingly precise information on the nature and consequences of gene damage caused by the plethora of environmental hazards that seriously threaten the quality of our life in the twenty-first century, and beyond, is becoming available. In the light of this, it may be possible to devise much more effective future environmental management strategies. Whilst these may not be sufficient to eliminate many of the problems that are already pressing on us, they nevertheless could help us achieve a far less toxic future than otherwise might be the case. We have already had many warning signals. This book aims to promote awareness of both the long- and short-term consequences that are likely to occur from an attack on genes either from environmental sources or as a result of some of our new gene technologies.

**Key points in this chapter**

- Even in the sixteenth century it was realized that all substances are potentially poisons and it is the dose that differentiates a poison from a remedy.
- By the eighteenth century it was recognized that exposure to chemical substances in the workplace can have adverse effects on those working with these substances. This formed the basis of occupational medicine and much workplace legislation.
- Despite these early warnings, we have created a diverse new chemical environment over the last two hundred years as a consequence of our industrial and agricultural activities.
- Many chemicals from the environment can enter cells and modify genes. In a number of cases these events can lead to the development of cancers. Other environmental hazards that can also damage genes and cause cancers include sunlight, nuclear radiation, and even food components.

# 2

# Genes – the targets of hostilities

The beginning of the new millennium saw gatherings of religious groups all around the world, hopeful of witnessing a second coming. In the event, the faithful were denied a holy reappearance. Moreover, there were no signs of any progress towards the eternal damnation of disbelievers, or even a Y2K bug. What did occur, however, around that time was the final and miraculous unravelling of the human genome in draft form. The human genome is the complete recipe of the genes that govern the way we are made and how we function. This deciphering was an extraordinary event, and the achievement is one of the most significant landmarks in human history, coming after a decade of intense effort by many researchers across the world. In 1919 Rutherford split the atom; in 1928 penicillin was discovered; the first heart transplant was carried out in 1967. The events at the turn of the century will have no less fundamental effects on the way in which medicine develops for hundreds of years to come. As long as we continue to exist, knowledge of the human genome will be important.

## The book of life

In a joint news conference held in June 2000 via satellite link, UK Prime Minister Tony Blair and US President Bill Clinton paid official tribute to all the researchers involved in what has been dubbed by some the Book of Life and others as the Map of Mankind. President Clinton referred to the achievement as the most important, most wonderful map ever produced by humankind. Completion of the rough draft of this book or map has also been described as the biological equivalent of putting a man on the moon. As explorations of space begin to reveal our true situation in the universe, so the human genome is revealing a great deal about our own origins and history on the earth. We may think we are very sophisticated, but already the map is showing us that we share countless genes with insects, worms and plants. Most of our genes are very like those of other animals; for example the genes of chimpanzees differ by only 1.5 per cent from those of man.

The actual process of unravelling the human genome developed into a contest that was often quite acrimonious. In many ways it was like the race of the tortoise and the hare, but without the predictable ending. Back in 1990 an enormous international collaboration began under the grandiose title of the Human Genome Project. US$3 billion was set aside to fund a programme that was then estimated as likely to take fifteen years. Things got up and running smoothly enough, and this consortium, mainly funded by the US government and Britain's Wellcome Trust, began the slow and methodical mapping of the genome with many of the sophisticated techniques that were then available. The comparatively relaxed pace of careful scientific progress carried out in the traditional way was, however, given a rude shock with the arrival on the scene of private entrepreneurship. A bitter race soon developed between the new boys on the block, Craig Venter and his Celera Genomics Corporation, set up in 1998, and the seemingly plodding, but solid and respectable, machinery of the global scientific establishment. In truth, Venter had been a part of the official effort, but left in 1996. Around this time, when working at the Institute of Genomics Research in the USA, he had developed a new and ex-tremely powerful technique for mapping genes and soon created a sensation by producing the first map of the genome of *Haemophilus influenzae*, a bacterium responsible for ear infections and meningitis. However, the effort required to produce this map was only equivalent to around a thousandth of that which would be necessary to produce a map of the human genome. His approaches cut out a lot of time-consuming chemical analyses, but were nevertheless greeted with con-siderable scepticism by the scientific establishment. However, within a brief time he was vindicated, and showed that, with his novel approach, he could probably shrink the timescale for mapping the human genome from years to months. A major component of his technique depended on the availability of massive computing power that was becoming available just around that time. As a further impressive demonstration of the power of his new approach, which dispelled any lingering doubts, Venter was soon able to release a CD-ROM containing a map of the genome of a fruit fly called *Drosophila*. With the equivalent of only thirty times more effort, the human genome map was in sight and Venter's techniques would probably deliver the goods. For his company he coined the phrase 'speed matters – discovery can't wait'. However, by the time of the dramatic announcements in 2000 regarding the 'first draft' of human genome, it is fair to say that the Celera Corporation had actually only mapped some 97 per cent of the human genome and did not expect to map the remainder for some considerable time. Similarly, the Human Genome Project scientists did not expect to publish a complete map until at least 2003. Despite the declaration of a truce, considerable feuding and controversy have occurred. Each group has disputed the other's results, although they closed ranks to claim equal honours when their achievements were announced in 2000. Much of the rancour between the two competing groups presently centres on the wider availability of the map. While the Human Genome Project group is committed to providing the information freely to all researchers that require it, Craig Venter's Celera Genomics Corporation aims to patent genes and sell the information to pharmaceutical companies. Although these matters remain to be resolved, there is good reason to believe that all these advances will have dramatic implications for humankind, and, in the future, will reshape many sectors of the world economy. However, it is fair to say that companies involved in further researching the human genome are not expected to make any real money from these discoveries for some years yet.

## What are genes?

Before proceeding to discuss the effects of hostile environmental elements on genes, we need some background information on the nature of genes and how they operate.

Along with all the other living organisms on earth, we have the capacity to reproduce. Our offspring resemble their parents more closely than any other human beings. This continuity of human characteristics from one generation to the next is called *heredity*. Parents endow their offspring with the necessary information encoded within basic units of inheritance called *genes*. The effects of genes are very wide-ranging. For example, they can dictate the colour of eyes and hair, as well as serving as fundamental determinants of learning, language and memory, which are essential to human culture. However, as will become clear from what follows, genes and their actions can be profoundly influenced by factors in our increasingly hostile and diverse environment.

Even in the nineteenth century, many human diseases, such as gout, colour blindness and haemophilia, were believed to be hereditary. In 1814 the British physician Joseph Adams was able to draw distinctions between *familial* diseases, which he believed to be confined to a single generation, and *hereditary* diseases passed on from generation to generation. The great Charles Darwin himself was highly intrigued by the evidence for disease inheritance, but, like his contemporaries, was quite uncertain about the possible mechanics of the process.

It was in the, perhaps unlikely, setting of a monastery garden in 1866 that the basic rules of heredity were established. Brno, a town in what is now the Czech Republic, rests in an agricultural area where crops and orchards were of considerable interest. Gregor Mendel entered the theological college there in 1843 and, following an unsuccessful period as a parish priest, attended the University of Vienna for a short time to train as a science teacher. Despite Mendel having a keen mathematical mind, this venture was also unsuccessful, although his tutors kindled his intense interest in plant variation. Returning to monastic life, his twin passions for gardening and mathematics were put to good use. In the monastery there was a traditional interest in plants and horticulture and there, in the monastery garden, Mendel began a series of experiments, using peas, that would bring new insights to the study of inheritance.

The experiments Mendel conducted were both highly systematic and on a grand scale, lasting over eight years and involving some 30,000 plantings. He chose to mate seven pairs of varieties of pea plants, and, from the outcome of these procedures, established a crucial feature of heredity. He found that individual plant characteristics do not blend with each other as one generation follows another. Instead, inherited characteristics are associated with some type of 'indivisible elements', which, although originally referred to by different names, are what we now know as *genes*. In 1865, only six years after the publication of Charles Darwin's *Origin of Species*, outlining the principles of natural selection, Mendel presented his own findings in a local journal of science. Although Darwin's work provoked intense debate, Mendel was forced to continue his labours in the garden, as his work was completely ignored. He did, however, send a copy of his paper to a fellow scientist, Carl von Naegli, who, possibly for reasons of jealousy, simply replied that the work was incomplete and unconvincing. Naegli even went as far as to suggest that Mendel try to produce hybrids from another plant, hawkweed. This was in the full knowledge that hawkweed hybrids were technically very difficult to produce, as Naegli himself had found to his cost over many years of effort. Sadly, in 1868 Mendel left his beloved gardens to take up an administrative role in the monastery as its abbot for the last sixteen years of his life. Even worse, years later, many of Mendel's papers were burned by the abbot who succeeded him. However, by a stroke of good fortune, thirty-five years after its publication, Mendel's seminal paper was eventually found and the importance of his work became immediately apparent. A cruel irony is that, had Charles Darwin been aware of Mendel's work, many of the acrimonious debates and controversy concerning the nature of natural selection proposed in *Origin of Species* might have been readily resolved.

Although the mechanics of heredity still remained obscure, physicians of the nineteenth century continued to gather further information about inherited human diseases. In 1897 Archibald Garrod became intrigued by alkaptonuria, a disorder that turns urine dark and sometimes leads to arthritis. Garrod suggested that, rather than being due to a bacterial infection, its origin was a congenital 'error of metabolism'. He proposed a similar explanation for the condition of albinism, where sufferers lack colouring pigment in their eyes and hair. Despite his linking of human metabolism with the laws propounded by Mendel, Garrod's far-sighted theories went largely unnoticed. Proof that many human diseases had a hereditary basis did not come until the latter half of the twentieth century, with detailed work on the gene defects that lead to diseases such as sickle-cell anaemia, muscular dystrophy and cystic fibrosis. Mainly this was because it was only then that the precise nature of genes was beginning to be understood.

A breakthrough came in 1943 with the experiments of a Canadian scientist, Oswald Avery, working at the Rockefeller University in New York on the properties of various strains of the pneumonia organism. Pneumonia then was a killer disease, and research on the causative agent was seen as a medical priority. Avery showed that the pneumonia bacterium could be changed from an innocuous to a highly dangerous variety simply by adding to the innocuous variety a solution of a substance known as DNA, which he had previously isolated from the dangerous type. In short, DNA from the dangerous variety had acted somehow to reprogramme the harmless type of bacterium.

*Deoxyribonucleic acid*, to give DNA its full name, had actually been known for some time. It was initially isolated in 1869 by a Swiss doctor, Friedrich Miescher, from the pus-laden bandages of wounded soldiers in the German town of Tübingen. He used some of the newly discovered aniline dyes to detect DNA in the pus cells. Although Miescher entertained thoughts that DNA might have some connection with heredity, because it could be found in all types of cell, other scientists at that time unfortunately did not share these convictions, and, because of this, he spent the rest of his life studying other subjects. Later, however, researchers such as Walther Flemming used other aniline dyes to stain and visualize microscopically the thread-like structures in cells containing DNA that would become known as *chromosomes*. The word 'chromosome' was coined as a consequence of the vivid colours that the aniline dye staining procedures produced, and is derived from *chroma*, the Greek word for colour.

Although the ground-breaking experiments of Oswald Avery showed that purified DNA could transmit hereditary traits from one bacterial cell to another, he had no idea what features of DNA enabled it to do so. The world had to wait until 1953 for a further discovery, which, in retrospect, was probably the most momentous revelation of the twentieth century. Another scientist with the conviction that genes were made of DNA was a young American, James

Watson. Originally from Indiana University he migrated to the Cavendish Laboratory at Cambridge University after a brief spell in Denmark. The Cavendish Laboratory had already become legendary in the world of physics. There, J.J. Thomson had discovered the electron and Ernest, Lord Rutherford had split the atom. At the Cavendish, Watson, then 25 and known to all as 'Jim', was thrown into contact with an English physicist, Francis Crick, then in his thirties. Before Watson's arrival, Crick had been looking for an important research project to which he could devote himself. He found DNA of considerable interest; in fact, a major factor in his abandoning physics for biology arose from reading a book by another physicist, Erwin Schrödinger, entitled *What is Life?* This book put forward the concept that genes were the key components of living cells and that, in order to appreciate what life is, it was essential to understand genes. Despite the slight age difference between Watson and Crick, they functioned superbly as a team, sharing a passionate belief that the answer to the structure of genes lay in understanding the structure of DNA. Watson was extremely down to earth, carried no airs, and did not stand on ceremony, but, above all, he valued Crick's deep insights and stimulating influence. In his frank and personal account of the unravelling of the structure of DNA, *The Double Helix*, Watson describes how the frontiers of knowledge were pushed forward in a close atmosphere of ambition, amid personal, intercollegiate and international rivalry (interspersed with the pursuit of au pair girls, winter sports and games of tennis). Their basic approach involved a combination of X-ray diffraction analyses and chemical model building. By 1953, and with the crucial help of X-ray crystallographers Maurice Wilkins and Rosalind Franklin from King's College, University of London, they had achieved their objective; but even Watson felt a little uneasy when Crick walked into a local pub, The Eagle, and announced to everyone within hearing distance that they had found the secret of life. Despite this unexpected reticence, James Watson and Francis Crick had made history; their structure of DNA was published on 28 February 1953. The significance of the structure was impossible to miss; it carries the genetic information for all forms of life on earth. Overnight they had changed the direction of biology. Individually, both went on to make further enormous contributions, particularly in the elucidation of the intricate

–A T G G C T A G T C A T G G T T G G A T C C T A G G G–
–T A C C G A T C A G T A C C A A C C T A G G A T C C C–

**Figure 2.1** A very short piece of a DNA molecule drawn to show the special partnering between the nucleotides (represented by their respective letters) on opposite strands

cellular mechanisms required for the decoding of the information contained within DNA molecules. Moreover, it was Jim Watson who was later at the helm during the early stages of the international Human Genome Project, described earlier.

All living organisms are composed of cells, each no wider than a tenth of a millimetre. Importantly, each cell in the body contains the same set of DNA molecules that make up what is referred to as the *human genome*. This is the blueprint for development from a single fertilized egg cell to a complex adult being, composed of more than ten million million cells. DNA molecules are extremely long, string-like substances. Thanks to the pioneering work of Watson and Crick we know that they are made up of two strands, each of which is made up of a series of units called *nucleotides* linked sequentially to one another, just like the links in a very long chain. There are only four types of nucleotide unit to worry about, and, for simplicity, the initial letters of their full names A, C, G and T (adenine, cytosine, guanine and thymine) are normally used to symbolize them. In Figure 2.1 it can be seen that where there is an A on one strand, this is always partnered with a T on the other strand. Similarly where there is a G, it is partnered with a C on the other strand.

A critical feature of the structure proposed by Watson and Crick was that not only were the strands partnered in a special way through their component nucleotides but also that the strands were intertwined with one another in the form of a 'double helix'. Every day, many years ago, as a young researcher at Glasgow University I passed a six-foot-high model of the DNA double helix standing in the hallway of the Biochemistry Department. The model only contained a dozen or so pairs of nucleotides; a minuscule fraction of what is contained in one of our cells. The component atoms were displayed in bright

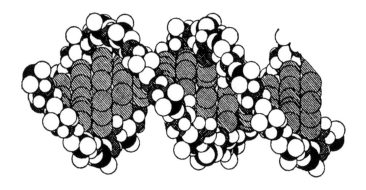

**Figure 2.2** A three-dimensional model of a
small segment of a DNA double helix

colours, black for carbon, red for oxygen, blue for nitrogen and white
for hydrogen, and there was a certain awesome beauty about the model
in its essential simplicity (see Figure 2.2). The DNA double helix
became an icon of the twentieth century. Its inherent simplicity in-
spires a deep sense of wonder, since from it emerges the miraculous
diversity and complexity of life on earth.

We share this extraordinary molecule with virtually all other life
forms. Although the sequence patterning of the nucleotide units varies
from species to species, the basic double-stranded structure of DNA
is universal: from moulds to molluscs, from bacteria to begonias, from
potatoes to primates, all rely on DNA to specify their form and
function.

When the arrangement of the nucleotides along the length of the
DNA strands is examined, it is clear that they are organized in very
precise sequences, just as letters of our alphabet are linked to form
words. The 'alphabet' of DNA, however, is more limited inasmuch as
it has only four letters, as compared with twenty-six. Despite this,
because individual DNA molecules are very long (some can be around
250,000,000 nucleotides, or letters, in length), they can carry a great
deal of information. Each individual DNA molecule within a cell
corresponds to a chromosome, which is effectively divided along its

length into segments referred to as genes. A simple analogy would be a cassette tape of the type you might purchase in a music store. The cassette contains a considerable length of narrow magnetic tape, which, although continuous, is effectively divided along its length into regions corresponding to the individual songs. Of course, the information corresponding to an individual song in the audiotape is encoded not in a sequence of nucleotides, but in a sequential array of variously magnetized particles. Like a chromosome, the audiotape is compactly wound within the cassette both for organizational purposes and to save space.

There are 46 DNA molecules, or chromosomes, in each human cell. Collectively, these are referred to as the *genome*. In reality, this represents two sets of DNA molecules. This is because one set of 23 distinct types is inherited from the mother and the other, similar, set of 23 from the father. To get some idea of scale, the smallest human chromosome is a DNA molecule of about 50 million nucleotide units linked end to end, whereas the largest contains around 250 million nucleotide units. If written out, the 3 billion letters representing all the nucleotides in a 23 chromosome set would fill two hundred 500-page telephone directories. If someone recited the sequence of letters at a rate of one letter per second, 24 hours a day, it would take a century to complete the reading. If you were able to extract all the DNA molecules from only one cell and then lay these molecules end to end, they would stretch for around six feet. It is an awe-inspiring fact that all these molecules are packed into a human cell of not more than a tenth of a millimetre across.

## Genes are blueprints for making proteins

Our bodies, like those of all other animals and plants, are formed from microscopic building blocks called *cells*. Cells are the fundamental unit of life, but very little would happen in cells without the participation of an important group of molecules called *proteins*. These are fairly large, three-dimensional molecules constructed within cells by the end-to-end linking of units called *amino acids*. It is the particular types of amino acid and the order of their linkage within a protein that determines its ultimate function. Basically, the information in a gene

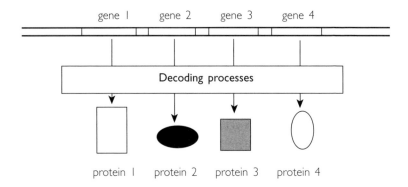

**Figure 2.3**  An illustration of a short piece of DNA indicating its subdivision into segments corresponding to four hypothetical genes, the information in which can be decoded to give rise to their corresponding proteins.

directs the selection of the amino acids, and the order in which they will be linked together to make up a particular protein.

To continue with our audiotape analogy, the sequential array of magnetized particles in a segment of audiotape is a code that specifies the progression of musical notes that go to make up an individual song. In a similar way, the sequence of nucleotides within a gene constitutes a code that specifies the precise order in which amino acids are linked within cells to create a single protein. A short piece of a DNA molecule is portrayed in Figure 2.3, with delineated regions corresponding to four hypothetical genes that are simply designated 1, 2, 3 and 4 for the purposes of the present argument. It is the information in these four genes that specifies the construction of proteins 1, 2, 3 and 4 respectively.

## What are proteins for?

Each gene carries the information necessary for the construction of a single unique protein, and since the DNA in each of our cells contains around 32,000 genes, it is not surprising there are many thousands of different proteins to be found within cells. Proteins are of fundamental importance, since virtually everything that cells do is dependent on the action of one type of protein or another. For example, a group of proteins help us to digest food and convert it into energy. Other proteins facilitate the functioning of senses and enable movements and thought processes, as well as contributing to reproduction and development. Still others serve as the basis of structures such as bones, cartilage or hair. The different capabilities of proteins depend on their shape and size, which, in turn, are a function of the order in which their constituent amino acids are linked together. Some can be quite large, but, on average, they are made up of between 100 and 1,000 amino acids. Quite simply, proteins are fundamental to life, which could not function without them.

## How are genes decoded?

Returning again to the analogy with the audiotape: without some sort of apparatus to convert the information held in its magnetized particles into recognizable music, the tape would be of little use. To decode a magnetic tape, an audiocassette player is required. As the magnetic tape passes over the playback head, the sequence of variously magnetized particles is translated into individual sounds that progressively make up the tune.

As already mentioned, a chromosome is a DNA molecule, which can be as long as 250 million nucleotides. Like an audiotape, this molecule can be subdivided along its length, not into segments corresponding to tunes, but into thousands of regions, or genes, each dictating the assembly of an individual protein along the lines illustrated in Figure 2.3. Although the length of individual genes can vary, the average is around 1,000 to 5,000 nucleotides. However, it is the specific sequential arrangements of the four nucleotides A, C, G and T along the length of a gene that determines the exact sequence in which amino acids will be liked together to create the protein specified by a particular gene.

All cells are equipped with intricate machinery, analogous to a playback head, to decode the sequences of nucleotides that make up each gene. This machinery is complex and involves the participation of another type of nucleic acid called RNA. Although a detailed appreciation of the cellular decoding apparatus is unnecessary here, the basic feature is that the process involves reading the nucleotides sequentially in groups of three at a time. For instance, the nucleotide sequence ATG in a segment of DNA specifies the inclusion of an amino acid called *methionine* into the protein under construction. Should a sequence TTC follow the ATG sequence in the DNA molecule, then an amino acid called *phenylalanine* will be linked to the *methionine* in the protein being constructed. If the next triplet of DNA nucleotides down the line is CAA, then the next amino acid to be linked up is *glutamine*. The process is continued step by step so that the sequence of nucleotide units in a gene is decoded to specify precisely the sequence of amino acids in a protein. This is the basis of the *genetic code*. Our technical abilities have advanced spectacularly, with the result that individual genes from humans and other living organisms can now be isolated, purified and the information in their individual nucleotide sequences readily decoded. The immensely long nucleotide sequences can now be fed directly into computers for detailed analysis. The Human Genome Project, which aims to establish the exact nucleotide sequences of all human genes, should probably be concluded by year 2003 and the sum total of the information accommodated in a couple of CD–ROM disks.

## DNA can be copied

Sixty years ago, we had only a very vague idea about the structure and function of DNA. Now we understand its elegance and simplicity, and the mechanisms by which it is decoded. A fundamental characteristic of DNA molecules is that their structure enables faithful copies to be produced.

As already mentioned, each of us starts life as a single cell (a fertilized egg); by the time we attain adulthood, we possess around 10 trillion ($10^{13}$) cells, each with a set of DNA molecules identical to the original set in the fertilized egg. This multitude of cells arises as a result of many cell divisions, in each of which a single cell gives rise to two offspring. In turn each divides to give two further progeny cells, and so on. Each of these cells, by an elegant copying mechanism,

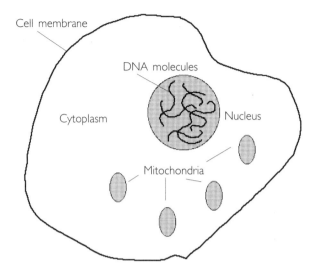

**Figure 2.4** A schematic outline of the structure of a cell

is issued with replicas of the DNA molecules that were present in the original fertilized egg. This copying mechanism is the way in which our children inherit our genes, from one generation to the next.

Microscopic inspection of a typical cell reveals the presence of a small blob-like structure, called the *nucleus*. This contains the *chromosomes*, or DNA molecules. In turn, the nucleus is suspended within fluid, or *cytoplasm*, which itself is surrounded by a membrane (Figure 2.4). There are many other structures to be found in the cytoplasm, for example *mitochondria*, used by cells for the generation of the energy that they require for their various functions.

In 1953, when Watson and Crick established the double-stranded helical structure of DNA molecules, they astutely commented that the way in which the nucleotides paired with one another in the opposite strands offered the basis of a copying mechanism. Because an A will always pair with a T and a G with a C, it is a simple matter to write out the nucleotide sequence of one strand, given the sequence of the other. This is precisely what happens each time a cell divides. Copying

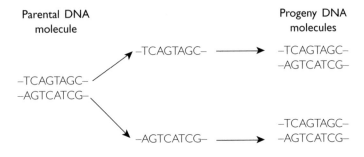

**Figure 2.5** The copying of DNA molecules. The separation of the two strands of a DNA molecule is shown, as well as the use of the separated strands, to guide the formation of new companion strands. The result is the formation of two double-stranded progeny DNA molecules identical to the parental DNA molecule.

of a cell's DNA molecules occurs at each cell division, so that each of the two cells that result inherits a replica set of DNA molecules (Figure 2.5). In complex mechanisms, facilitated by proteins within the cell, the two strands that make up a DNA molecule are effectively separated. The next step is that the nucleotide sequence of each separated strand is used as a guide for the formation of a new companion strand (Figure 2.5).

Although DNA is copied in cells with remarkable precision, very occasionally the insertion of the wrong nucleotide can occur – for example, a T is inserted, rather than a C – or sometimes bits simply fail to get copied at all and are therefore missing from progeny molecules. Fortunately, such mistakes occur extremely rarely during the normal copying process; somewhere in the region of only once for every million nucleotides copied. Nevertheless, these natural mistakes account for some of the variations encountered in the DNA from different individuals.

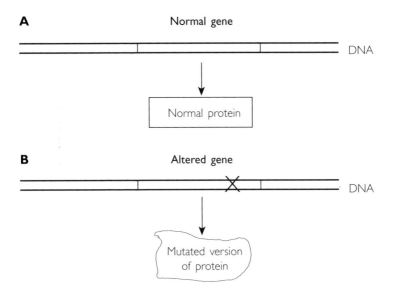

**Figure 2.6** The effect of an alteration in the nucleotide sequence of a particular gene on the protein normally produced by that gene. **A** represents the normal situation and **B** the situation after an alteration has occurred within the nucleotide sequence of the gene. The region harbouring the altered nucleotide sequence is represented with a cross.

## Mutations and their consequences

The linear sequences of nucleotides in DNA are not inviolate. Damage can cause alterations to the sequential arrangement of nucleotides in a segment of DNA corresponding to a gene. This is illustrated schematically in Figure 2.6. As will become evident in later chapters, a very large range of toxic environmental factors can bring about such damage, and a major problem occurs when the cell makes attempts to decode the altered sequence of nucleotides.

In the case of our audiotape, damage to the arrangement of the magnetic particles would be readily detectable on playback as a defect in the music emitted by that particular segment of the tape. Similarly, an altered DNA nucleotide sequence within a gene would specify a fault in the amino acid sequence of the particular protein normally specified by that gene. Because of its faulty amino acid sequence, this protein is said to be *mutated* and may no longer be able to carry out its proper function. The presence of such a variant, or *mutant*, protein can have serious consequences. For example it could bring about the development of cancers, or limit lifespan, or could be the basis of diseases inherited by our children.

## From egg to adult

In the mother's womb, a fertilized egg divides initially to produce two cells and then four and so on. During what is called *development*, many successive rounds of cell division follow, first producing an embryo, and then specialized cells, ultimately leading to a complex adult. Since each cell has 23 pairs of DNA molecules (or chromosomes), each progeny cell receives replicas of all 46 chromosomes. This is the way most cells divide, but in the cells of ovaries and testicles a somewhat more elaborate form of cell division occurs. Rather than having the usual 46 chromosomes, *eggs* or *sperm* cells are produced with only 23 chromosomes. However, when an egg with 23 chromosomes is fertilized by a sperm cell, the normal total of 46 is achieved again. In short, each one of us gets a set of 23 chromosomes from our father and another 23 from our mother. In the ensuing chapters of this book, sperm and egg cells are referred to as *germ cells*, whilst the remaining cells that make up the bulk of our bodies are called *somatic cells*.

## Genes and the environment

The similarity of humans as a whole, from one generation to the next, arises out of the overall general correspondence of the genetic blueprint that is repeatedly followed in their construction. Although variations between individuals in the human population arise from small differences in the genes that make up the general blueprint, it is also clear that the environment can have a profound effect on the ultimate outcome. The combined influences of genes and the environment have been well appreciated for some time by biologists observing the development of plant and animals. In the case of humans, the embryo is carefully maintained in the controlled conditions of the mother's womb. However, if this delicate environment is altered, abnormalities in the way the embryo forms can result. For instance if a mother drinks excessive levels of alcohol, or suffers German measles during pregnancy, or takes drugs such as thalidomide, the child can be born severely malformed.

While the complete array of genes in an individual determines the potential of that person, the characteristics actually realized depend on the interaction of these genes with the environment. These characteristics unfold during the complex processes of development and maturation from egg to adulthood when genes, and the products derived from them, interact with one another and the environment. A characteristic cannot be solely attributed to genes or the environment. *Successful survival requires the interplay of both.* Individual genes provide the initial guidelines for development and a range of possible outcomes. Within a predetermined range, set by an individual's genes, the final outcome is shaped by environmental influences.

Each cell contains the same molecules of DNA. These contain genetic information equivalent to around 32,000 genes, but not all these genes are active in every cell. Despite this, a small proportion of genes are in fact active in almost all cell types and are sometimes referred to as the *housekeeping genes*. Primarily they encode proteins that are normally required by all cells, regardless of type, just in order to keep them ticking over. Such proteins may be involved, for example, in basic processes such as energy production or utilization of oxygen. In contrast, other genes are only active in cell types that require the presence of particular proteins in order to carry out their specialized functions. For instance, in muscle cells the genes encoding muscle proteins such as *actin* and *myosin* are switched on, whereas in liver cells these proteins are not produced, and other genes, such as the one for making the liver protein *albumin*, are active. Neither the muscle protein nor albumin genes are active in brain cells. There, other genes encoding proteins required for brain function will be switched on.

Even if a gene is present in DNA, it may be inactive, or switched off. Many proteins are actually only required under certain conditions and regulatory systems that function as on–off switches allow them to be produced as and when required. Other, more refined, mechanisms can make minor adjustments in the levels of particular proteins, in response to needs imposed by the environment. In addition, when a gene is switched on, the protein it produces has the potential to interact with other elements within the environment of the cells, as well as external environmental factors, such as dietary components and temperature. For example, we have genes that are important for the digestion of sugars and are sensitive to the presence of sugars. In the cells of the intestine these genes can be switched on specifically in response to sugars taken in the diet. Increases in temperature can also switch on a number of genes to produce proteins whose job it is to help cells survive the stress of excessive temperature fluctuations. These particular genes have sometimes been referred to as the *stress genes* and can also be switched on during viral infections, or in response to the presence of poisonous metals from the environment such as arsenic, cadmium, lead and copper, or certain toxic drugs and environmental chemicals. We also have genes that can be activated to provide some protection for our cells in situations of oxygen deprivation, excessive ultraviolet radiation or exposure to substances called free radicals. These aspects will be expanded upon in later chapters.

How, then, are genes switched on or off depending on the special requirements of different cell types? Close inspection has revealed that not all the nucleotide sequences in DNA actually encode proteins. Certain sequences lying outside the coding regions of genes form part of the switching mechanism whereby the activity of specific genes can be adjusted. Not only do nucleotide sequences in DNA determine precisely the type and structure of the proteins made by cells, they also comprise part of the machinery that controls the level to which these proteins are produced in response to cell requirements. In the same way there are also sequences associated with other genes that allow them to be switched on or off in response to different environmental conditions (Figure 2.7).

When it comes to dealing with very complex human characteristics, such as behaviour and learning, the interactions between heredity and the environment are really much too complicated to be properly understood at the present time. Despite this difficulty, we know that there are human gene defects that can be inherited and that are associated

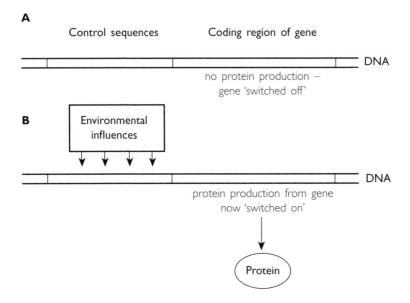

**Figure 2.7**   The general layout of a gene whose activity is influenced by the environment. A shows the situation in the absence of environmental influences, and B illustrates the situation in the presence of environmental influences.

with behavioural abnormalities, although the connections are difficult to explain in terms of gene activity at present. For example, the inherited disease *porphyria* stems from a defect in one of the genes that controls the proper assembly of the red-coloured pigment in blood cells. This pigment is responsible for carrying oxygen from the lungs to the tissues. Among the symptoms exhibited by sufferers of porphyria is the production of discoloured urine. Another, perhaps surprising, symptom is periodic bouts of mental instability. Medical history suggests that King George III, the unstable British monarch of the late eighteenth century, suffered from porphyria; the film *The Madness of King George* portrayed how the disease may have affected him mentally. Other descendants of Mary Queen of Scots also suffered episodes of madness, and her son King James VI produced urine the colour of wine, suggesting that they too suffered from this disorder.

Mental retardation is a characteristic of another inherited human disease, *phenylketonuria*. This condition is caused by a fault in a gene that directs the construction of the protein responsible for the normal breakdown of the amino acid *phenylalanine*. The faulty protein that results cannot carry out its normal function, phenylalanine cannot be broken down and accumulates excessively in body fluids and, under certain conditions, can be converted to compounds that can lead to brain damage. The Lesch–Nyhan syndrome is also due to an inherited fault in a gene. In this case, the gene in question is responsible for directing the assembly of a protein involved in producing the basic components for the building of DNA. Although the connection is not yet clear, sufferers from this disease compulsively bite and mutilate their fingers and lips.

It is clear that alterations to genes can profoundly affect human behaviour in ways that we are far from understanding. It seems very likely that environmental factors will also affect such genes. Until we understand genetic influence on behaviour much more thoroughly than at present, a full evaluation of the effects of environmental stresses will be very difficult.

---

**Key points in this chapter**

- The continuity of human characteristics from one generation to the next is termed *heredity*.
- The basic units of inheritance are *genes*.
- Genes are specific segments of extremely long string-like molecules of DNA, made up of only four units called *nucleotides*, linked together in a vast variety of different sequences.
- Each gene directs the construction of a protein using a decoding mechanism that reads the *genetic code* in sequential groups of three nucleotide units.
- Errors in the nucleotide sequence of a gene can lead to the assembly of faulty, or *mutant*, proteins. Such errors can be caused by certain hazardous environmental factors.

- An identical 46 (23 pairs) DNA molecules, referred to as *chromosomes*, reside in the nuclei of all cells (except eggs and sperm which have 23).
- At each cell division, the DNA molecules are copied so that each progeny cell inherits a replica set.
- Errors in the copying process do occur naturally but at an extremely low frequency.
- *Development* refers to the complex processes that lead from the fertilized egg to adulthood and that can be influenced by environmental conditions.
- Whereas the complete set of genes of an individual can set an individual's potential, the final characteristics of that individual depend on the interaction of their genes with the environment.
- The environment can profoundly influence the activity of many genes. Alterations to genes can change human behaviour; it is likely that environmental factors are also capable of causing such changes.

# 3

# Nuclear attack

For much of the twentieth century, security has taken precedence over environmental considerations. By far the worst offenders in this context were military–industrial complexes, especially those involved in the nuclear weapons business. Driven by the need to end the Second World War, as well as by the intellectual excitement surrounding the then recent discoveries of the fundamental forces binding atoms, the atomic bombings of Nagasaki and Hiroshima were the culmination of intense research efforts by American and British physicists in the 1940s. Shortly after 8 o'clock in the morning of 6 August 1945, an object fell earthwards from *Enola Gay*, a B29 Superfortress bomber piloted by Col. Paul Tibbets. Soon the falling object became a searing flash of light and energy and, by evening, the Japanese city of Hiroshima and 71,376 of its people no longer existed. That moment of massive destruction and loss of life marked the end of an era for physicists – at that moment they forfeited their innocence. Another atomic bomb devastated Nagasaki three days later, and, although the war ended in another four days, by the following summer quite a number of those involved had turned their backs on the troubled world of nuclear physics. Fortunately, some looked towards biological problems. This union of physics and biology was particularly successful in establishing the structure of DNA, as outlined in the previous chapter. The X-ray crystallographers Francis Crick, Maurice Wilkins and Rosalind Franklin – who sought to apply a number of physics-based techniques to important biological phenomena – were all physicists.

Since the end of the Second World War, everyone has been exposed to unnaturally high levels of nuclear radiation. The superpowers competed with one another to make more and more powerful nuclear bombs. The USA built tens of thousands of nuclear warheads and, in the process, billions of gallons of radioactive waste material were released into rivers. As a result, some of this water penetrated ground waters. Fifty years or so of weapons production in the USA left huge amounts of radioactive waste, including much that is very long-lived. This has proved expensive and technically difficult to eradicate, and, even today, only a partial clean-up is possible. The Soviet nuclear programme was similarly environmentally irresponsible. Initiated by Stalin, it produced weapons as fast as possible. This was simply to match the US progress and was done with no regard to human or environmental costs. They built some 45,000 warheads and dumped the bulk of their nuclear waste at sea, mostly in the Arctic Ocean, some of which is quite shallow. For reprocessing spent nuclear material they used the Mayak complex on the Ob river in western Siberia. This is still the most radioactive place on the planet. From 1948 until 1956, the complex unloaded its radioactive waste into a tributary of the Ob, which was then the sole source of drinking water for the surrounding population. In 1957, a storage tank actually exploded, releasing large amounts of radioactive material into the atmosphere. After 1958, liquid waste was stored in Lake Karachay, but, in 1967, because of a prolonged drought, winds were able to spread the resulting radioactive dust over an area reputed to be nearly the size of Belgium, to a level of activity some 3,000 times that encountered at Hiroshima. Unfortunately, most of the radioactive material persists until the present day, because the current Russian administration cannot afford an effective clean-up.

The awesome properties of nuclear weapons were continuously demonstrated by tests carried out in the open air. Radioactive fallout from the familiar mushroom clouds quickly became dispersed over the earth's surface, driven by prevailing winds and rainfall systems. The USA is reputed to have tested over 1,000 warheads, and the USSR around 715, in the years between 1949 and 1991. During that time, the Soviets even used nuclear explosions to create reservoirs and canals as well as opening mineshafts. Although large-scale releases of radioactivity from such sources have become less of a problem in recent times, another potential hazard has grown in importance. Since the

1970s, there has been a growing dependence in a number of countries on nuclear fission as a source of power for the generation of electricity. At present there are around 400 nuclear power plants worldwide. Initial publicity promised a source of electricity that was safe, clean and cheap. On the contrary, there is now evidence to indicate that nuclear power is highly unsafe, being capable of polluting on a massive scale, as well as proving extremely costly. Public opinion now seriously questions the safety and the future growth of the nuclear industry, particularly in light of the increasing age of most of the installations, together with the legacy of the horrific accidents at Three Mile Island in the United States in 1979 and at Chernobyl in the Ukraine in 1986.

## Nuclear weapons

It is now almost a century since the physicist Ernest Rutherford discovered the nucleus of the atom. By 1911, he had shown that most of the weight of an atom was located in this unimaginably small object at the centre of the atom. Within the nucleus, enormous energies lie trapped; these are the basis for two developments that have had profound impacts on our way of life: nuclear weapons and nuclear power.

By the late 1930s, scientists had discovered most of the principles behind nuclear energy and how these could readily be applied. The outbreak of World War II elicited fears that Germany might choose to develop nuclear energy for military purposes. This concern fuelled the development of nuclear weapons by teams in the United States and Great Britain. Although the name *atomic bomb* has been widely used for more than a half century, a more accurate term would be *nuclear bomb*. This is because the energies released by nuclear weapons arise not from atoms as such, but from the nuclei within them.

After his discovery of the *atomic nucleus*, Rutherford found that it could be shattered by high-energy bombardment. In 1932 another British physicist, James Chadwick, discovered the *neutron*, one of the building blocks making up the nucleus. Although the Italian physicist Enrico Fermi found that it was possible, by bombardment, to add extra neutrons to existing nuclei, making them heavier, some very unstable situations resulted. To regain stability, some of these over-weight nuclei can shed components to yield lighter nuclei that are more stable. When this occurs spontaneously it is referred to as *radio-active decay*. On the other hand, when extra neutrons strike an already massive uranium atom, there is a high chance that it will split apart into large pieces. This process is called induced *nuclear fission*. In addition to fragments arising from this break-up process, there are many neutrons produced. These can go on to induce the break-up of other uranium nuclei. In this way, a *chain reaction* is possible in which one uranium nucleus induces the fission of two adjacent uranium nuclei, which in turn induce the fission of four other uranium nuclei. The net result is a cataclysmic process in which most of the nuclei in a piece of uranium would fragment and release inordinate amounts of energy. *Nuclear fusion* of hydrogen nuclei also releases massive amounts of energy, but requires great amounts of heat to initiate the process. Both fission and fusion bombs have been produced, with the latter requiring the extreme heat from a fission bomb to initiate the explosion.

Following the explosion of a fission or fusion bomb, a prodigious number of nuclei and other nuclear components are released, travelling at enormous speeds. These readily collide into atoms and molecules in the vicinity, creating a fireball of enormously high temperatures as well as causing massive radiation damage to nearby areas. The explosion also generates a burst of burning light that includes all the components of the electromagnetic spectrum: infrared and microwave radiation, visible light and ultraviolet radiation and radio waves as well as gamma and X-rays.

*Fallout* is much less spectacular, but much more insidious, and is a consequence of both fission and fusion explosions. It involves the generation and liberation of *radioactive substances*. The fission of plutonium and uranium creates products that are still relatively unstable. These products emit high levels of radioactive radiation, albeit at very different rates. Some become harmless after millionth parts of a second, yet others can endure for millions of years.

## Nuclear power

A nuclear power station harnesses the energy released in a controlled chain reaction of nuclear fissions of unstable uranium or plutonium in an enclosed reactor. The fission reactions release energy that can then be extracted as heat by a circulating cooling fluid such as water. It is this heated fluid that is then used to generate electricity. A new generation of reactors has been mooted that would be based on the energies released by nuclear fusion. At the moment, however, such reactors remain at the development stage.

Providing energy for an increasingly hungry, developing world is an extremely complex problem with no easy, risk-free, environmentally friendly solutions readily available. Although the use of nuclear energy has some attractions, increasingly the hazards of even low-level environmental contaminations are being seen as outbalancing the benefits. Genetic effects of the resulting radiation are a critical aspect when risk assessment is being undertaken.

## Problems of radiation

Life has evolved on earth in the face of radiation of many kinds. Most of these radiations come from the sun, but others arrive from outer space and some from the rocks of the earth itself. Some, such as visible light, are essential for life, being trapped by plants that, in turn, serve as a source of energy for the growth and multiplication of other living organisms. In contrast, the radiations arising from radioactive elements in the earth or the cosmic rays from space are not essential for life, and, in many cases, are potentially harmful. Fortunately, they occur at only very low intensities, and living organisms on earth are well adapted, at the present time, to cope with their effects.

Although we have always been exposed to radioactivity, its existence was only appreciated as recently as a century ago. In 1895, Wilhelm Röntgen, while investigating the properties of electric discharge through cathode ray tubes, discovered a new type of radiation. He was a shy, secretive experimenter who normally worked alone in a laboratory in Würzburg, Germany. His investigations involved examining the effects his newly discovered rays had on photographic plates. Soon, he found that he could use them to produce 'shadow pictures' of the interiors of various objects. Six weeks after his initial discovery he persuaded his wife to have her hand photographed using his newly discovered rays. The result was a blurred but recognizable image of the skeleton of her left hand, with her ring visible as a dark band on the bones of her fourth finger.

The nature of these new rays that could penetrate soft tissue was puzzling to scientists at that time. Because a magnet could not deflect them, they were unlike the then well-known cathode rays. Nor were they light rays. Because he could not fully understand them, Röntgen opted simply to call them *X-rays*. The general public were immediately mesmerized, and popular magazines soon appeared with pictures of Röntgen himself together with X-ray pictures of fish and frogs, revealing their delicate skeletons.

Shortly after Röntgen's discoveries, another French scientist, Henri Becquerel, found that a somewhat similar type of radiation was emitted by ores of uranium; and Pierre and Marie Curie isolated radium, a substance that is highly radioactive. Indeed, the dangers of radium soon became apparent when Becquerel burnt himself as a result of carrying some in his pocket. Taken together, these events defined two important properties of the new type of radiation. Not only could it penetrate living tissues but it could also kill them. Such properties found almost immediate application in the field of medicine. X-rays were very soon being used to examine the internal organs of living patients, and the rays from radium to kill the cells of malignant tumours. In fact, diagnostic and therapeutic radiology, as these approaches became known, are still very much in use today.

Unfortunately, these new, beneficial technologies had associated risks. In the rush to establish the new techniques, the early radiologists ignored certain clear warning signs. These included symptoms such as severe dermatitis occurring on the hands that they used to throw a shadow on a screen when testing the beams of X-rays. In time, this dermatitis developed into ulcers and then, after a number of years, to cancer, from which most of the pioneer radiologists died. Although in retrospect it all appears foolhardy, it has to be remembered that the development of tumours at that time was poorly understood. As will be discussed later in this book, we now know that cancer development can often take up to twenty years; the initial dermatitis probably seemed relatively innocuous at the time. An equally subtle hazard came to light from work carried out in 1928 by geneticist Hermann J. Muller, then at the University of Texas. In his laboratory he exposed fruit flies to large doses of X-rays and induced impressive numbers of mutations in their genes. Muller's flies still looked and acted the same after their radiation treatments, but many of their offspring certainly looked different. It was soon apparent that radiation posed a hazard not only for those exposed but also for their descendants in successive generations. In 1956 Alice Stewart, a British clinician then at the Oxford Institute of Social Medicine, discovered that even a single dose of diagnostic X-rays shortly before birth will double the risk of an early cancer death for a newborn child.

These studies indicated that it was essential to determine what risks were entailed in exposure to varying amounts and differing kinds of radiation. In addition, it was important to work out how best to use radiation, not only to minimize the harm but also to maximize the therapeutic benefits. Today, many stringent rules and regulations govern the use of and exposure to radiation. These rules are far from perfect and are still the subject of much heated debate.

## What exactly is radioactivity?

When the nucleus of an atom undergoes spontaneous disintegration, there can be a radiation of energy and/or pieces of the broken nucleus. These radiations are what we refer to as *radioactivity*. There are quite a number of substances occurring naturally with atoms that have unstable nuclei and can spontaneously release radioactive radiations. Additionally, there are many man-made substances that can also release radioactive radiation. The *alpha*, *beta and gamma* radiation released by the nuclear disintegration processes carry a great deal of energy and are dangerous because they can take electrons away from other atoms. This results in the formation of *ions*, and is the reason why they are often referred to as *ionizing radiations*. Another form of radiation capable of ionization is X-rays.

There is a lot of variation in the penetrating powers of these different forms of radioactive radiation. Gamma rays, as well as X-rays, are extremely energetic and it takes several centimetres of lead shielding to block their passage. In contrast, beta radiation can barely penetrate human skin, and a sheet of paper can easily stop alpha radiation.

## Safety from nuclear radiation

At present, nuclear reactors are built with multiple layers of safeguards and the release of radioactivity into the environment is usually small, although large quantities of waste can be produced. This has raised serious problems with regard to its handling and long-term storage. Some of the radioactive waste will remain hazardous for hundreds of thousands of years. Nowhere in the world has the nuclear industry really been able to show that it can deal safely with these highly dangerous wastes. Despite protestation that nuclear reactors, unlike the systems that produce electricity from coal burning, would limit atmospheric pollution, nuclear facilities, as presently operated, will contaminate our environment for the foreseeable future. Although it was originally envisaged that the long-lived radioactive waste products would simply be disposed of deep underground, this was an inadequate solution. A severe limit on the amount of new waste needs to be seriously considered. Over the world as a whole, there are already radioactive wastes equivalent to around a thousand times that released in 1986 from the core of the reactor at Chernobyl in the Ukraine. The bulk of these wastes will have to be completely isolated from the environment for centuries to come, unless we can find a safer way to dispose of them. Reprocessing, which separates plutonium and uranium from spent nuclear fuel, has been considered as a possible approach. One disadvantage is that the reprocessing process is extremely expensive. Additionally, the products may have a limited market, as various countries are now seriously reviewing their commitment to nuclear power in light of hostile public opinion. There is, of course, still the possibility that the products of reprocessing could be marketed for the development of further nuclear weapons.

Since the end of World War II, when mushroom clouds became a familiar sight, our planet has been systematically irradiated as a result of radioactive fallout from nuclear tests, as well as accidental discharge of radioactive wastes from nuclear reactors. In the parts of the world where cancer registries kept data, the rates of childhood cancers and leukaemias were found to have risen, particularly in the period that began twenty years after the 1955 to 1963 era of intense fallout from weapons testing. This delay before rates increased is probably very significant. As will be explained later, the development of most cancers is a long-term process, often taking between fifteen and twenty years from the initial exposure to the cancer-causing agent. In areas of the UK, such as Wales, where the fallout was highest, the onset of these cancers began just slightly less than twenty years after exposure.

By 1970, as a result of nuclear fallout, most people had the radio-active substances plutonium and strontium in their bodies. Although the testing of nuclear weapons had been gradually phased out in the 1960s, the hazards from radioactivity did not diminish. Instead of bombs, both controlled and accidental releases from nuclear power stations and reprocessing plants took over as a source of radioactive pollution of the biosphere. A very worrying feature was the apparent clustering of leukaemia cases in the vicinity of these nuclear plants. By the 1950s, the Irish Sea became a dumping ground for considerable amounts of low-level radioactive waste from the Windscale plant at Sellafield in Cumbria. Although much of our normal waste is routinely dumped at sea, this radioactive waste did not simply disappear from sight. Instead, many radioactive substances attached themselves to mud and silt particles, which, under the influence of maritime currents and tides, resurfaced later as components of estuarine and harbour mud flats. Continuous wave activity also caused some of the smaller radio-active mud particles to become airborne. As a consequence, significant quantities of low-level radioactive particles were propelled for considerable distances over land.

It is important, nevertheless, to put these issues in some proper perspective. The levels of radioactivity we are likely to be exposed to from these sources are 100 to 1,000 times lower than those suffered by survivors of the nuclear blasts at Hiroshima and Nagasaki in 1945. Those survivors, of course, were sufficiently distant from the explosion not to be completely incinerated or suffer complete tissue and cell breakdown. Exposure to very high levels of radioactivity simply kills cells. Exposure of humans to high but non-lethal levels of nuclear radiation will induce radiation sickness (skin burns, hair loss, nausea and loss of immune function), but lesser exposure can still cause mutations as well as damage to bone marrow, spleen, lymph nodes and blood cells, together with long-term problems such as infertility, neurological damage and cancers.

What is a safe dose of radiation? While the survivors of the Japanese explosions were exposed to relatively high levels of radiation, this was mainly in the form of a single external dose. In contrast, one of the problems with our long-term exposure to the radioactive products of fallout from weapons testing, or reactor failures and the wastes from reprocessing plants, is that relatively low levels of such products can still be readily inhaled or ingested. This creates the situation of exposure from internal rather than external sources. For instance, particles containing the radioactive substance plutonium 239 can pass from inhaled air through the membranes of the lungs, and be caught in lymph nodes, where they continue to emit alpha rays that can massively irradiate surrounding tissues and their DNA molecules, potentially leading to cancers. Despite the tiny dimensions of some particles, they have the ability to locate at critical tissue surfaces. Another radioactive substance, caesium 137 (an emitter of both beta and gamma rays) has an affinity for muscle and liver tissues. Iodine 131 (also an emitter of beta and gamma rays) concentrates in thyroid glands and promotes the development of thyroid cancers, which are notably increased in the survivors of the Chernobyl accident. Ruthenium 107 (yet another emitter of beta and gamma rays) can locate in the bone marrow and wreak havoc with the formation of blood cells in a way that may ultimately lead to leukaemias. Another concern is that some products of nuclear fallout and reprocessing plants can imitate and take the place of natural nutrients. For example, our bodies will accept strontium 90 (a beta ray emitter) in place of calcium, which is a normal component of bones, and is also routinely found associated with DNA of chromosomes. Because of this ability to mimic calcium, airborne strontium 90 deposited on grasslands becomes concentrated in cows' milk, and is readily ingested as part of the normal diet. When associated with chromosomes in place of the normal calcium, it can bring about damage to DNA.

Another product that is often neglected, but that can also cause gene damage, is the radioactive form of hydrogen called tritium. This can take the place of normal hydrogen atoms in a wide range of molecules, including DNA. A problem arises as the nuclei of tritium atoms disintegrate. Not only are beta rays emitted during this process but the tritium atoms also change their identity to helium atoms. Such helium atoms, in the place of the normal hydrogen atoms, can damage the structure of the afflicted DNA molecules and lead to mutations.

Despite these concerns, which are very real for those living in the vicinity of nuclear reactors or reprocessing plants, of the *average* total radiation dose that most people are exposed to at the present time only about 0.5 per cent actually arises from nuclear plant emissions and nuclear weapons testing. In contrast, as much as 10 per cent is unavoidable, coming from outer space in the form of *cosmic radiation*. This background radiation from space is the 'flash' of the Big Bang that heralded the creation of the universe some fifteen billion years ago. It is observed in every direction within space and is the lingering signature of creation.

Although diagnostic medical X-rays account for roughly another 12 per cent of our radiation exposure, of more concern is the radiation that arises from uranium that occurs naturally in rocks and soils. Direct radiation from this source accounts for about 14 per cent of the average radiation exposure, but a more insidious problem is *radon*, which, in certain situations, can represent as much as half the average annual exposure. This colourless and tasteless gas is a product of the decay of the uranium in rocks and soil, and hazards arise because it can readily seep into the basement areas of buildings, where it accumulates if the ventilation is poor. It has been estimated that radon may account for as many as one in twenty lung cancer deaths in the UK.

## How does ionizing radiation damage genes?

As already mentioned, alpha, beta and gamma rays, as well as X-rays, carry a tremendous amount of energy and are dangerous because they can take electrons away from atoms to form ions. This process is called *ionization*; hence these radiations are usually referred to as *ionizing radiations*. Because approximately three-quarters of the mass of most cells and tissues is water, around 75 per cent of the ionizations produced in irradiated cells occur in water molecules. Some of these water ions are unstable and undergo reactions, either spontaneously or in collision with other molecules within cells, to yield stable but highly reactive entities called *free radicals*.

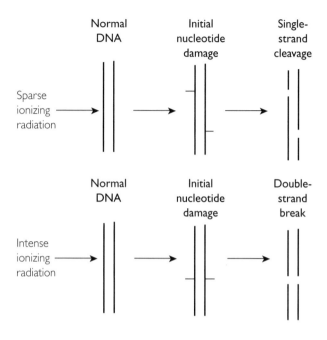

**Figure 3.1**    Radiation-induced breakages of DNA strands

Ionizing radiation can damage molecules in cells in two ways: first, by direct action involving the ionization of cellular molecules themselves; second, by indirect action where water molecules are first ionized, and then generate reactive free radicals, which subsequently damage cell molecules such as DNA. The comparative levels of direct and indirect damage to molecules within irradiated cells and tissues are usually difficult to assess. This is because, within cells, some molecules are simply physically isolated from water, while others are effectively protected by a screen of substances that have the property of reacting preferentially with free radicals.

DNA is particularly vulnerable to assault by free radicals, which are reactive by virtue of a deficiency in electrons. Various bits of the DNA nucleotide units are susceptible to free-radical attack in different ways.

Initially, this can lead to structural damage to nucleotide units, and, sometimes, to the breakage of the individual DNA strands themselves. Because DNA has two strands, cleavage of only one of them does not disrupt the molecule as a whole, and, if randomly distributed, many such cleavages can accumulate before the DNA collapses into two or more pieces. The free radicals generated by sparse ionizing radiations probably cleave only one DNA strand at a time, without causing the DNA molecule to break apart. In contrast, more intense ionizing radiations are more likely to sever each DNA strand at the same, or nearly the same, point, thus causing a *double-strand break*, which will lead to the molecule breaking into discrete parts (Figure 3.1).

A considerable body of opinion now implicates double-strand breaks in DNA as the major underlying cause of *cell death* after irradiation. In comparison, DNA nucleotide modification and single-strand cleavages brought about by ionizing radiations appear to be of less significance in relation to cell death. They are more likely to be critical in relation to the *mutations* that can be induced by ionizing radiation. Very low doses of radiation can induce mutations. Indeed there appears to be no threshold below which mutations are not induced by ionizing radiation.

## Clinical uses of ionizing radiation

Despite the inherent safety issues, ionizing radiation has applications in clinical medicine. With stringent precautions and limitations, X-rays are used in two situations: imaging and radiation therapy. In *X-ray imaging*, the rays are passed through the patient's body to a sheet of photographic film, or an X-ray detector. Although most of the X-rays pass through the tissues, bones block some of them. In this way the patient's bones create a shadow image on the film behind. *Radiation therapy* also uses X-rays, but to kill cancer cells. However, to attack and destroy tumour tissues deep beneath the skin, much higher energy radiation has to be used than is the case for imaging. It has also been found in practice that DNA double-strand breaks and cell killing by intense radiation can be enhanced by the presence of oxygen. Unfortunately, a feature of many tumours in the human body is that, unlike normal tissues, they receive only poor supplies of oxygen. This can limit the effectiveness of any radiation therapy. Because of this, there have been a number of attempts to develop drugs that can be given to patients to improve the oxygen levels in their tumours, and thus enhance the killing power of the X-rays.

---

**Key points in this chapter**

- Nuclear explosions from weapons based on either nuclear fission or fusion generate very high temperatures and massive amounts of radioactivity. Fallout is a significant hazard.
- Reactors used to generate domestic electricity utilize controlled nuclear fission. Problems exist with the safe disposal of radioactive waste that can be hazardous for many years.
- Radioactivity is the radiation released when the nucleus of an atom spontaneously disintegrates. Because of its properties, it is referred to as ionizing radiation.
- Ionizing radiations are dangerous because they can damage the DNA of genes in various ways, resulting in mutations in some cases. High levels of exposure to ionizing radiations can kill cells, a property used as the basis of anticancer therapies.

# 4

# A phoney war?

Although the threats from ionizing radiation are very real, there is a growing tendency to see risk everywhere. Should we still watch television? Is it safe to use hairdryers considering our close proximity to their heat and electromagnetic fields? How far back should we stand whilst heating up our chips in the microwave?

One of the most widely publicized of such concerns is the electromagnetic radiation from mobile telephones, computers and electricity pylons. The possibility has been raised that these may be a health hazard, and could also lead to the development of cancers. This may simply be a symptom of the neurotic times we live in, but on the other hand some caution may be advisable.

The widespread use of mobile phones is a recent phenomenon, with a significant escalation over the last decade. For many they are an essential part of business, commerce and society, and it is likely that their use, together with related technologies, will continue to increase for the foreseeable future. There has been much public debate about possible adverse effects on human health. It has been established that use of mobile phones while driving increases the risk of road accidents by causing lapses in concentration. However, more subtle concerns have centred on the radiations emitted from the handsets themselves, and from the base stations that receive and transmit the signals.

## Electromagnetic radiation

The complete spectrum of electromagnetic radiation includes radio waves, microwaves, ultraviolet radiation, visible light, infrared radiation, gamma rays and X-rays. Our eyes detect only a very small section of this spectrum that corresponds to *visible light*. This particular section has a wave length that lies between 400 and 700 nanometres (a nanometre being a millionth of a metre), on a scale of wavelength that varies between ten metres, which is the wavelength of AM radio, and less than a nanometre, which is the wavelength range in which we find gamma-rays and X-rays. In Chapter 1, the harmful properties of the ultraviolet components of the sun's radiation, with wavelengths between 280 and 400 nanometres, were alluded to in connection with the induction of skin cancers. Both nuclear radiation and sunlight are acknowledged to be major health hazards; a question now asked is, how do they compare in terms of health risk with the radiations from mobile telephones, as well as microwave ovens and electricity pylons?

Mobile phones undoubtedly emit electromagnetic radiation, but so do television and radio transmitters, as well as microwave ovens. On the other hand, we are likely to be in very much closer contact with mobile telephones than with radio transmitters and microwave ovens. In the case of hand-held phone use, the exposures to radio frequency radiation will be principally to the side of the head.

As well as the worries about mobile phones themselves, there is also disquiet concerning emissions from the base stations that make up the phone network. In general, exposure from these will be to the whole body rather than just the head, but the levels of intensity experienced will be many times less than those from handsets. Base stations communicate with phones within a defined area usually referred to as 'cells'. These come in many shapes and sizes. *Macrocells* have a power output of tens of watts and constitute the main structure of a network, with an ability to communicate with mobile phones over a range of up to about 22 miles. There are currently around 20,000 such cells covering the country, with the number set to increase. At the moment, measurements indicate that exposures of the general public are typically many hundreds, or thousands, of times lower than the existing exposure guidelines set by the National Radiological Protection Board in 1993. Despite this, it may be that emissions from all base stations may not be uniformly low, and, with the predicted increased use of mobile phone technology, there may yet be an unacceptable increase in the level of emission. *Microcells* are used to infill and improve the network and are located, for instance, at airports, railway stations and shopping malls. These emit much less power than macrocells, with a range of only a few hundred yards. Provided the protective case surrounding the antenna remains in place, there is little chance of overexposure from microcells. Finally, *picocells*, usually located within buildings, have an even lower power output still.

## Possible effects of mobile phone technology on DNA and human health

The radiations from phones, microwave ovens and television and radio transmitters range in wavelength from around 50 millimetres to about 5 metres, but they have an extremely high frequency. Unlike the low frequency ionizing radiation of gamma rays and X-rays, high frequency microwave radiation does not have enough energy to cause any ionizations, break chemical bonds or damage DNA directly. Because of these properties, the microwave radiation from mobile phones is very unlikely to cause *direct* damage to our DNA. For the moment, however, this does not rule out *indirect* effects on DNA that might be a consequence of interactions of high-frequency radiation with other cell components that, in turn, could produce secondary-damaging agents such as free radicals (see Chapter 3). Another possibility, recently mooted, is that mobile phone radiation indirectly causes DNA damage to accumulate, simply by impairing our normal DNA repair systems (described in Chapter 9). Experiments in which experimental rats and mice have been exposed to microwave radiation have, so far, failed to demonstrate any convincing evidence for increased cancer rates, but, for reasons that will be discussed later in this book, the timescale of such animal experiments may be insufficient. Moreover, other possible radiation effects such as local microwave heating should not be discounted prematurely. However, compared with a microwave oven, a phone has only a thousandth of the power, and, if you feel your ear heating up when making a call, it is most likely to be either the batteries and electronic circuitry heating up, or just the embarrassing nature of the conversation, rather any direct radiation effect.

Yet another possibility is that, whilst not causing any significant local heating, microwave radiation from handsets may interfere with the subtle electrical interactions between cells that are involved in the maintenance of nearby brain tissues. This could possibly affect important functions, such as memory and other cognitive processes. Conceivably, non-thermal effects could also interfere with the normal regulation of growth and interactions of brain cells. As will be explained later, loss of cell growth control is extremely relevant to the long-term development of cancers.

In 2000, in a far-sighted move which sensed public apprehension, the Executive of the Scottish Parliament set up an Independent Expert Group under the chairmanship of Sir William Stewart to report on the 'Possible Effects of Mobile Phone Technology on Human Health'. In May 2000, the Group submitted its report, in which it stated that it is not yet possible to say that radio-frequency microwave radiation, even at levels below the present national guidelines, is totally without health effects. In short, there are still too many gaps in our knowledge to be sure, and the group wisely urged a cautious approach. In itself, this was a momentous step. In the past, very little cautionary advice regarding potential environmental hazards was given to the public until it was almost too late. Hopefully, this advice from the Expert Group will put some brakes on the excessive use of mobiles, particularly by children, whose skulls are not yet fully thickened and are likely to be using phones for much longer periods than adults.

On balance, the task of proving scientifically that the microwaves from mobile phones are *absolutely harmless* is likely to be impossible. For instance, it is impossible at this time to give mobile phones a clean bill of health regarding cancers, because cancers can take up to twenty years to develop, and mobile phones have simply not been in general use for enough time to make a definitive judgement. Although the 'jury is still out', there was a study in 1999 led by Lennart Hardell from Sweden in which the fates of 209 patients diagnosed with general brain tumours were compared with a matched group of 425 healthy subjects. He was unable to find any overall increased risk of brain tumours among those who used mobiles. However, he did observe that a very small group of cellphone users were about two and a half times as likely as non-users to suffer tumours in the lobes of the brain adjacent to their 'phone ears'. Since this group comprised only 13 patients, the observation could readily be dismissed as a statistical artefact. More extensive studies over a long period, with larger numbers of subjects, are still required. Additionally, the Swedish study was based on the use of analogue phones; digital phones could easily be more harmful. The latter use pulsed microwaves, and their power could increase five-hundredfold during the dialling processes. More definitive data on the possibility of cancer development may take another ten years to produce. However, it may be wise to consider such information as a warning signal, and, for the moment, the precautionary approach seems very prudent because we do not really know what the long-term effects may be. Already, manufacturers of mobiles have begun to use 'smart' antennas and other means to lessen the exposure of callers to microwaves. Putting up the costs of calls is, of course, another approach.

Public apprehension about electromagnetic radiation does not stop with mobile telephones. Electromagnetic fields occur in the vicinity of television and radio masts, overhead power lines and electricity substations, household appliances such as electric blankets, burglar alarms, VDUs and microwave ovens, as well as the electronic tagging devices used in shops to prevent theft. As already pointed out, microwave radiation does not cause ionizations, as is the case for gamma rays and X-rays. Instead, the major problem with non-ionizing microwave radiation is its ability to generate localized heat. At the very high strengths generated in microwave ovens, the heat created within the irradiated food is sufficient for thorough cooking. By comparison, many low-level microwave radiations are incapable of causing any perturbations whatsoever. This, however, leaves open the question of potential hazards from intermediary levels of radiation. Worldwide, there are reports from people living near mobile phone transmission masts of fatigue, sleeplessness, anxiety and short-term memory loss. These effects are unlikely to be due to heating, as the intensity of the radiation from the radio masts is too low. As with the mobile phones themselves, there may be some more subtle electrical effects that are perpetrated possibly at the level of nerve cell function. On the other hand, such symptoms could be caused by other factors in the environment.

In light of the recommendations of the Stewart Independent Expert Group mentioned above, the Scottish Executive passed legislation in 2001 that makes it more difficult for mobile telephone operators to erect masts wherever they like. As a result, Scotland is now the most tightly regulated place in Britain for ground-fixed mobile phone masts, but, predictably enough, the Scottish business community immediately complained that the country was becoming a 'wireless backwater'. However, at the beginning of 2002 the UK government launched a £7.4 million research programme, lasting three years, aimed at providing definitive answers on the safety, or otherwise, of mobile phones. Fifteen separate research projects will investigate a wide variety of possible biological effects from mobile phone radiation. A further four studies will seek to determine whether the use of mobile phones increases the risk of brain cancer or leukaemia. Others will look at the effect of mobile phone signals on body function and examine how the body absorbs the energy. This research, which is also backed by the mobile phone industry, should go a long way towards ending the confusion that currently surrounds the safety of mobile phones and masts.

## Power lines and pylons

Epidemiological studies have suggested that living near high-voltage power lines *might* increase the risk of childhood leukaemia, but only by a factor of 1.5 to 2. Despite the very weak statistical evidence for a link between power lines and leukaemias, there is nevertheless public concern that radiation emitted from these lines can have adverse effects on human health. Overhead power lines are known to attract water droplets containing high concentrations of atmospheric pollutants, some of which are known to cause lung cancers. The radioactive gas radon that occurs naturally in the atmosphere (as mentioned in the previous chapter) is also attracted by power lines. It arises from the normal decay of uranium present in rocks and soils. Radon, however, is known for its ability to cause lung cancer, rather than childhood leukaemias. Moreover, a recent large-scale statistical study that actually involved going into homes to measure electromagnetic fields failed to find a link with childhood cancers. Besides measuring the fields generated indoors by household wiring and electrical appliances, these studies also took account of input from any nearby power lines. Whatever the cancer risk from electromagnetic fields in the home, it appears too small to detect. As is the case with mobile telephones, such studies certainly do not guarantee absolute certainty, but it would be useful to seek alternative explanations for the childhood cancers.

---

**Key points in this chapter**

- Mobile phones, microwave ovens, radio and television transmitters all emit high-frequency electromagnetic microwave radiation.
- High-frequency microwave radiation does not have sufficient energy to damage genes directly, although the possibility of indirect damage should not be discounted.
- Mobile phones only have a thousandth of the power output of a microwave oven.
- Although the possibility that the use of mobile phones might cause brain cancers or other health effects exist, it is simply too early to give a definitive view one way or the other, and a precautionary approach to their use is recommended.
- There is weak statistical evidence for a link between pylons and electric power lines and human cancers. Power lines can attract water droplets containing high levels of atmospheric pollutants. However, recent measurements of electromagnetic fields in nearby houses have so far failed to substantiate links with cancer, but such studies cannot yet guarantee freedom from risk.

---

# 5

# Chemical attack

Almost forty years ago Rachel Carson's *Silent Spring* warned of the impact of chemicals on the environment. No single book on our environment has done more to awaken and alarm the world. It arose from Carson's frustrated attempts to become a professional marine biologist at a particular time when women were notably unwelcome in the academic community. Her views concerning the potential dangers of synthetic chemical pesticides in the environment took shape during her time in various relatively low-level government posts, as scientist and editor. She was a courageous ecologist, but, most importantly, she became an influential nature writer. Her determination to speak out and save the natural world she adored resulted in the publication, by the late 1950s, of three brilliant and popular books about the sea. This was during the early days of the Cold War, when the possibility of global extinction was frighteningly real. She completed *Silent Spring* in 1962 in the face of almost overwhelming odds, confronting a US government and industry that seemed to be recklessly putting the future of the world's living species at risk with large-scale industrial pollution. Despite challenging and changing the prevailing culture of her time, the world does not yet seem sufficiently alarmed. Her scientific, but passionate, exposure of the effects of the indiscriminate use of chemicals is still very relevant today. The argument that, unless we recognize that human beings are only a part of the living world, our progressive poisoning of the planet will end in catastrophe, remains a classic statement.

We should not have been surprised or caught unawares by *Silent Spring*. A clear link between an environmental chemical and cancer was reported over 220 years ago. As already mentioned, this was thanks to the perceptiveness of Percival Pott, a London physician. He was puzzled by an unusual incidence of sores located on the scrotums of many young chimney sweeps in his local area and reasoned that the chimney sweeps were really afflicted by a type of skin cancer. He argued that men, such as chimney sweeps, continuously exposed to irritants in soot were especially likely to develop this type of cancer. Today we now appreciate that the presence in the soot of a chemical called *benzpyrene* was to blame. A hundred years after Dr Pott revealed his remarkable insight, physicians in Germany and Scotland noted skin cancers in workers whose skin was in constant contact with tar and paraffin oils that we now know contain *polycyclic aromatic hydrocarbons* (PAHs). In 1895, it was observed that aniline dye workers in Germany were prone to the development of urinary bladder cancers. Comparable findings were later made in a number of countries and a possible relationship was established between exposure to three chemicals (*2-naphthylamine, benzidine* and *4-aminobiphenyl*) and bladder cancer. What is notable about these pioneering discoveries, linking environmental chemicals and cancers, is that they were made on human subjects, without the use of experimental animals. Nowadays, much of the work to test the safety of environmental chemicals in this context is done using experimental animals. In 1915, the first successful attempt to induce cancers in animals involved the repeated application of coal tar to the ears of rabbits, with the resultant production of skin carcinomas. Using this approach, it was finally possible to identify the active cancer-causing agent in coal tar as benzpyrene. Much work was subsequently done in the 1930s to identify other synthetic chemicals that could also cause cancers in experimental animals. Liver cancers were induced in rats and mice with *dimethyl aminobenzene,* and urinary bladder cancers in dogs with 2-naphthylamine. The list of known cancer-causing chemicals expanded in the 1940s, with the discovery of *acetyl aminofluorene* (AFF), *halogenated hydrocarbons* and *urethane.* Since the 1940s, many other synthetic chemicals have been added to the list, including various *nitrosamines* and *vinyl chloride.*

Since the Industrial Revolution, we have created an extraordinary chemical environment. At that time, steam power became the paramount source of energy. Fossil fuels such as coal, oil and natural gas are still burned today in massive amounts, releasing bizarre chemical cocktails into the air we breathe, the water we drink, and the soils we use to cultivate our food. The petrochemical industry uses these same fuels to create the raw materials for synthetic consumer products such as plastics, paints, dyes, pharmaceuticals, cosmetics, food and food additives. Each process releases waste chemicals into the environment, and, when the products are used, they themselves are excreted, dumped or burned, thus adding to the general burden of synthetic chemicals in the environment. Such chemicals also arise during aluminium, iron, steel and coke production as well as in rubber manufacture. A further source has been the industrialization of agriculture, necessary to support the growth of urbanized industrial societies. This latter activity is highly dependent on the use of fertilizers and pesticides at high levels for intensive cultivation, as well as the extensive use of pharmaceutical products in livestock husbandry. Such practices add to the high levels of synthetic chemicals in water and soil, together with residues in the food chain.

In recent times, we have become more and more concerned with the role that manufactured chemicals can play in the processes that lead to the development of major human diseases, particularly cancer. Many industrial processes that are known to give rise to occupational cancers involve exposure of workers to specific synthetic chemicals. For instance, polycyclic aromatic hydrocarbons are generated in aluminium, iron, steel and coke production, and *aromatic amines* in the rubber and dyestuffs industries. Over time, aromatic amines were added to rubbers and cutting oils to act as accelerants and anti-rust agents. Despite the compelling studies carried out on dogs in the 1930s, which clearly indicated the potential of these chemicals to cause cancer, aromatic amines such as the *benzidine dyes* remained in commercial use for a further forty years. They were used not only in industries such as leather, paper and textiles but also in situations where the general public would be exposed, beauticians and craft workers for example. Although by 1994 benzidine was no longer commercially available in the USA, it could still be detected in chemical waste sites, in sediments of water systems and in the air, associated with small particles.

If such chemicals in the environment play a significant role in cancer development, it should be the case that high incidences of the disease are to be found in locations where these chemicals are concentrated. Such areas would include the industrial sites of manufacture, or waste sites where they might be dumped. Up until the end of World War II, such chemical waste sites did not exist. However, that was the moment when consumer products such as plastics, detergents and pesticides, together with all the undesirable by-products of their manufacture, began to make a significant appearance, and chemical waste dumping became an environmental problem. The incidence of a variety of cancers has been found to be higher than normal in populations exposed to contaminants at waste sites.

Anyone born after World War II thus belongs to the first genera-tions to grow up in relatively close proximity to high concentrations of man-made chemical refuse of almost unlimited diversity.

There is now an unprecedented range of synthetic compounds, produced for industrial and agricultural purposes, that are released into the environment, and that have no clear relationship with chemical compounds already in the natural world. In this context, it is im-portant to realize that, besides the molecules that make up both human beings and other living organisms, the natural world also contains a diversity of compounds produced, or excreted, by these organisms. Additionally, chemicals are created by naturally occurring long-term geological processes, for instance coal, petrol and natural gas. Petroleum oils arise from the accumulation of residues from algae and bacteria in shallow seas and contain paraffins and compounds like benzene, to-gether with many other chemicals. Coal, in contrast, is mainly derived from land-based plant matter, and comprises complex polycyclic sub-stances, as well as a variety of sulphur-containing compounds.

Microorganisms, such as the bacteria and fungi of soils and ground water, have coexisted for many millions of years with such naturally occurring chemical compounds. In fact, microorganisms play a funda-mental role in the global recycling of matter, mainly due to their metabolic versatility. They particularly excel at utilizing naturally occur-ring organic waste in soils and ground water as sources of energy and nutrition. In the process, they conveniently eliminate these sources of potential environmental pollution. Natural communities of fungi and bacteria in soils and water are normally made up of highly complex and interdependent groups. Waste chemicals are usually efficiently broken down in such environments, since the range of degradative possibilities is probably greater in a community, and products produced by one organism in the community are quite likely to be utilized by another organism. Overall, the combined activity of several organisms may lead to the complete degradation of the waste compounds to carbon dioxide and water. In practice, an important application of this versatility of microorganisms is in the routine treatment of sewage and other waste water, to remove substances that might be a health hazard.

In contrast, substances released into the environment, but with no obvious relationship to chemicals already in the natural world, are usually difficult to eliminate, as their breakdown in the environment is extremely slow, often taking many years. Such compounds are usually referred as *xenobiotics*. Many are released as components of fertilizers, herbicides and pesticides. Others, such as polycyclic aromatic hydrocarbons and *dioxins*, are products of combustion events. Dioxins result when attempts are made to eliminate garbage and medical wastes by incineration. Other xenobiotics are detectable in waste effluents resulting from the production and use of synthetic chemicals. A hazardous aspect of a number of these xenobiotics is that they can become progressively more concentrated with every step in the food chain. Striking examples of such xenobiotics are *polychlorinated biphenyls* (PCBs) and *phthalate esters* (plasticizers for cellulose and vinyl plastics). PCBs have wide applications, including use as hydraulic fluids, plasticizers, lubricants, flame-retardants and dielectric fluids. Although their manufacture was halted in 1977, their degradation in the environment has been agonizingly slow.

The years since 1945 have seen a dramatic increase in the rate at which novel synthetic compounds have been created. It has been estimated that there are now around 75,000 synthetic chemicals in common use, a significant number of which appear to cause cancers, and against which we have no natural protection. Safety procedures and protective legislation have slowly evolved for the workplace. Unfortunately, it is not just industrial workers that are exposed. Such massive amounts of chemicals are now produced and used that they are no longer contained within the workplace, but are slowly seeping into the environment, due to their release into air and water from toxic waste dumps, accidental spills or farm runoff. Many xenobiotics such as PCBs and pesticide residues find their way into food; in fact they may now be said to be basic contaminants of our food. Moreover, our children tend to receive higher doses of any xenobiotics in the air, water or food, since they breathe, eat and drink proportionately more than adults. *Organochlorides*, such as the pesticide *DDT*, are highly persistent in air and water. They become deposited as a result of winds and storms in the soil and vegetation, and from there enter the food chain, so that our diet is probably the main route of exposure. Although DDT and PCBs were banned in the 1970s in most countries, both can be detected in human tissues to this day. By 1951, DDT-contaminated human breast milk was passing the chemical from mother to child. In our tissues, we convert much of the DDT to another compound, *DDE*, which appears to accumulate with age, especially in fatty tissues.

Many animal studies have shown links between chemical compounds and cancers. In the wild, as graphically illustrated in Rachel Carson's *Silent Spring*, animals inhabiting contaminated environments have often developed cancers; and, in the laboratory, many synthetic, as well as natural, compounds will induce cancers in experimental animals, particularly rodents. With the exceptions of the connections between scrotal and skin cancers and coal tar, and tobacco smoke and lung cancer, precise links in humans have been more difficult to establish, although it is very reasonable to speculate that aromatic amines are linked with bladder cancer and *phenoxyherbicides* with non-Hodgkin's lymphoma.

## Some synthetic chemicals can modify DNA

Not surprisingly, there is now intense interest in the various ways in which different synthetic chemicals can alter the structure of DNA. Inevitably, with such an immense array of chemicals it is difficult to know where to begin. In the event, it has only been possible to investigate the actions of a relatively small number at the present time. Regrettably, the first significant studies on the interactions of synthetic chemicals with DNA arose from the notion that man-made chemicals might be useful as the basis of lethal weapons in warfare. A good example is *mustard gas*, first developed by Germany as a chemical warfare agent in World War I.

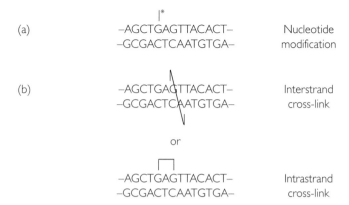

(a) | -AGCTGAGTTACACT-<br>-GCGACTCAATGTGA- | Nucleotide<br>modification

(b) | -AGCTGAGTTACACT-<br>-GCGACTCAATGTGA- | Interstrand<br>cross-link

or

-AGCTGAGTTACACT-<br>-GCGACTCAATGTGA- | Intrastrand<br>cross-link

**Figure 5.1** Various modifications to DNA that can occur following attack by different types of synthetic chemical: (a) the modification * of a single nucleotide unit, (b) the creation of a cross-link between nucleotide units on the two opposite strands of a DNA molecule (interstrand cross-link), or the formation of a link between two nucleotide units within the same strand of a DNA molecule (intrastrand cross-link).

Despite the relative shortage of detailed information, it is clear that some chemicals are a problem because they can enter cells and directly damage the structure of DNA nucleotide units. One group, examples of which are nitrosamines and vinyl chloride (a precursor of the plastic *polyvinyl chloride*, or PVC) do so by chemically adding part of themselves to single nucleotide units of DNA so as to create a modified version (*) of that unit as illustrated in Figure 5.1(a).

Unlike these examples, there is another group of chemicals with structures that allow them to react with DNA at two sites simultaneously. If the two sites are on opposite strands of the target DNA molecule, this can lead to the formation of *interstrand cross-links*; conversely, if the two sites are on the same strand of a DNA molecule, then the result is an *intrastrand cross-link* (see Figure 5.1(b)). The former variety of cross-links is especially problematic; they prevent the separation of DNA strands during the processes of DNA copying for future cell progeny. As a result, these chemicals are particularly toxic as they ultimately prevent normal cell division. Because of this, a number of chemicals capable of creating interstrand cross-links have

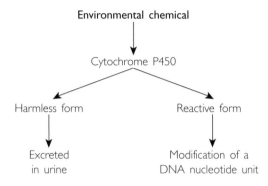

**Figure 5.2** The transformations of an environmental chemical
by cytochrome P450s

been put to use clinically as therapeutic drugs aimed at stopping the
proliferation of undesirable cancer cells. Examples of these are the
drugs *cyclophosphamide* and *cis-platin*.

Yet another group of environmental chemicals can pose a threat
when they are changed within cells to more reactive forms that are
able to modify DNA nucleotides. Chemicals in this group, which
includes polycyclic aromatic hydrocarbons, are transformed by a group
of proteins in cells collectively referred to as the *cytochrome P450s*. Paradoxically, the normal function of these particular proteins is actually to
*protect* us from the adverse effects of toxic environmental chemicals
and drugs. They do this by converting these potentially toxic chemicals to forms that are soluble in water, and capable of being got rid
of in urine. This is what usually happens, but sometimes the structure
of some synthetic chemicals in the environment is such that the process
of transformation, instead of producing a harmless version of the
chemical, gives rise to highly reactive, potentially harmful forms that
now have the ability to modify DNA nucleotide units directly (see
Figure 5.2).

As a specific example of this sequence of events, we can look at
benzpyrene, originally detected in coal tar, but later found in cigarette
smoke and car exhaust fumes. Cytochrome P450s can transform
benzpyrene to *phenols* and *dihyrodiols*, which can be safely excreted in

urine. Unfortunately, in addition to these harmless products, some unpleasant *reactive epoxides* can also result. These can join up with certain nucleotide units of DNA molecules to cause bulky modifications, usually referred to as *adducts*.

## Cytochrome P450s

The cytochrome P450s are very diverse and appear to have evolved in response to a variety of environmental challenges in our distant past. It is estimated that there are between 60 and 200 different types of cytochrome P450, divided into ten different families. At present we know that three of these families are responsible for reducing the potentially harmful effects of environmental chemicals such as drugs, organic solvents, anaesthetics, dyes, pesticides, alcohols, odorants and flavours. Whilst the P450s have a clear role in the defence of cells from the ravages of such toxic chemicals, their Jekyll and Hyde character must not be ignored. Although they can protect, they nonetheless are able to convert certain types of seemingly innocuous chemicals into extremely reactive forms, capable of modifying DNA. It is now clear that different people have considerable heritable variation in their complement of cytochrome P450s. Thus, individuals will show variation, compared with others, in their ability to deal with various environmental chemicals, in their transformation either to harmless or to destructive variants. In short, the susceptibility of humans to the newly created chemical environment is likely to show considerable variation.

## Bad air

In recent times, humankind has managed to wield exceptional power over the atmosphere that provides a canopy of support for all life on earth. This canopy is a surprisingly thin, gassy layer that surrounds the planet. It is only around 100 kilometres from top to bottom and, in comparative terms, weighs only 0.0003 per cent of the water that makes up the world's oceans. This makes the atmosphere very much easier to pollute than the seas. Although nitrogen and oxygen are now the predominant gases of the atmosphere (78 and 21 per cent respectively), there are also many other gases present, but often only in trace amounts. Two of these other gases have gained some notoriety in recent times, namely ozone and carbon dioxide.

Before the twentieth century, the only serious atmospheric pollution arose from cities; this was mainly due to smoke and soot arising from the burning of fuels like coal, peat and oil derived from plant material. As the century rolled on, so the pollution cocktail became more complex. This was especially so by the 1960s, when automobile exhausts challenged the emissions from chimneys and smoke stacks. By 1990, road traffic had become the largest single source of pollution around the world. Car exhaust contained many pollutants which contributed to the generation of *smog* and *acid rain*. Another serious atmospheric pollutant, after 1923, was lead, which can induce a range of clinical symptoms in both adults and children. The introduction of lead into the atmosphere was mainly due to the efforts of Thomas Midgley, an American chemical engineer. He discovered that it was possible to make petrol burn more effectively and, at the same time, reduce engine 'knocking' by the addition of lead. For the next fifty years cars around the world were propelled by leaded petrol. Although there was a great deal of alarm at the time lead was introduced into petrol (and even a governmental inquiry), General Motors and Dupont together managed to avert any regulation of lead additives in the USA until the 1970s. By that time, lead levels in the blood of most Americans were seriously elevated, but in 1975 it became mandatory to sell low-lead petrol in the USA. Western Europe followed suit in the 1980s, and other countries by the 1990s. This legislation reduced the levels of lead in the US atmosphere by 95 per cent by 1994, and the blood levels in American children also fell. The levels of worldwide atmospheric lead contamination are, however, still far from ideal. From the 1970s, cars became more fuel-efficient and new technologies became available for reducing noxious emission from exhaust pipes, but, unfortunately, pollutants still spew forth. Indeed, around a quarter of the carbon dioxide added to our atmosphere comes from automobile exhausts.

## Oxygen can be bad for us

The high concentration of oxygen that eventually built up in the earth's atmosphere after Precambrian times was due to the activity of photosynthesizing bacteria and plants. They harnessed the energy from sunlight to provide the necessary food for their existence using light-dependent processes that involved taking in carbon dioxide and water and giving out oxygen as a by-product. Although most forms of life are dependent on oxygen, in certain circumstances it can be a mixed blessing. In the stratosphere (10–30 km above sea level) the effect of the sun's radiation on oxygen produces the *ozone layer*, without which, as will be explained in a later chapter, relatively few organisms on the planet would be able to survive. This is 'good' ozone, but there is also 'bad' ozone nearer the ground.

Ozone was very fashionable in the latter part of the nineteenth century. People used to flock to the seaside to breathe in 'the ozone'. This all contributed to the successful commercial development of many seaside resorts. However, the smell of the seaside is actually nothing to do with ozone. Today you are more likely to get a small whiff of ozone using the underground on the way to the office, or from the photocopier once you get there. Rather than promoting health, ozone is actually bad for us; very small amounts can cause breathing difficulties, and it can also damage vegetation. Whilst lightning generates some ozone, the bulk of the bad ozone near the ground, and which we breathe, arises from sunlight acting on pollutants in smog, which is now highly prevalent in modern cities with large numbers of car users. Strong sunlight acting on oxygen, and emissions from car exhausts at ground level, favour the generation of various reactive free radicals, as well as ozone. Unlike the ozone of the stratosphere, this ground-level ozone is a health hazard. Later, in Chapter 8, we shall return to some of the environmental issues surrounding ozone.

## Burning plants

### Carbon dioxide production

For many thousands of years, humankind has burned plants to provide warmth and to cook food. In more modern times, we have taken to burning fossil fuels, derived from ancient plants, on a massive scale. Such burning of coal and oil not only consumes oxygen, but also produces carbon dioxide from their hydrocarbon components. Carbon dioxide is now accumulating in the atmosphere at an unprecedented rate. Since the Industrial Revolution, atmospheric levels have increased by some 30 per cent and the present level is set to double by 2050. Whilst this may be good news for plants, which take up carbon dioxide, such inappropriate changes in atmospheric levels of carbon dioxide are likely to affect the delicate natural balance of atmospheric gases that is required to maintain the correct greenhouse effect. Warmth from the sun heats the earth's surface, which then radiates energy, some of which is trapped by water vapour and carbon dioxide in the atmosphere. This trapped radiation is important as it warms the earth's atmosphere close to the surface. The 'greenhouse effect' that is created is very critical for keeping the earth's surface comfortably warm, and for the maintenance of life, as we know it. On the other hand, small increases in the concentrations of greenhouse gases, such as carbon dioxide, can have dramatic effects on global temperatures and weather conditions. In addition to carbon dioxide, other gases can also contribute to the greenhouse effect and global warming. These include methane, nitrous oxide and ozone, as well as *chlorofluorocarbons* (CFCs), perhaps better known for their ability to deplete the stratospheric ozone layer (see Chapter 8).

The plants from which fossil fuels are derived contain nitrogen and sulphur components, in addition to the more abundant hydrocarbons. Their combustion thus also releases oxides of nitrogen and sulphur into the atmosphere. On top of this, there are likely to be products of partial combustion such as volatile organic compounds, as well as particulate material.

## The creation of nitrogen oxides

Automobile exhaust is a major source of *nitrogen oxides*. In general, the composition of nitrogen oxides in the atmosphere is complex and they are involved in many different reactions influenced by light, temperature and local concentration. Mainly, they are formed when nitrogen in fuels or combustion air is heated above 650 degrees Celsius. Besides automobile exhaust, other sources of nitrogen oxides include power stations and various industrial processes. Bacteria of soil or water, which utilize nitrogen-containing compounds for energy, also contribute nitrogen oxides. Although nitric oxide is usually produced first in the above situations, this is readily converted in the atmosphere to nitrogen dioxide. It is this reddish brown gas that gives smog its colour and can damage our lungs. Nitrogen oxides can also combine with water to give nitric acid, a major component of acid rain.

## Particles of soot

In addition to nitrogen oxides, sulphur dioxide, carbon monoxide and a mixture of incompletely burned compounds, automobile exhaust also releases particles of soot with highly toxic properties, a particularly rich source being diesel exhaust. This is a hazard of growing importance, especially due to the increasing truck traffic in middle Europe, following the opening up of the east. The particles are quite small and can be easily breathed in. Crucially, they have carbon cores with a large surface area onto which a very large variety of compounds such as PAHs, aromatic amines and metal atoms, such as iron, can be absorbed. The particles can cause mutations and cancers in experimental animals; although it is not yet clear which components are to blame, obvious possibilities include the PAHs and aromatic amines. However, the presence of iron may also promote the formation of free radicals, which, in turn, may cause much damage to nucleotides units of DNA.

## Sulphur dioxide production

The burning of fossil fuels, especially cheap low-grade coals of high sulphur content, is a major source of atmospheric *sulphur dioxide*. As well as causing long-term respiratory problems, it is a contribution to the possible development of lung cancers. The replacement of coal with cleaner domestic heating fuels has reduced emission in the UK since 1970 by around 60 per cent. There are also natural sources of atmospheric sulphur dioxide such as volcanoes, sulphur springs and the weathering of minerals, as well as from the activity of microbes. Sulphur dioxide is a problem for us, as it readily dissolves in water and the fluids of tissues, and gives rise to sulphite and bisulphite ions, as well as related free radicals that can damage DNA nucleotides and bring about breakage of chromosomes. Bisulphite ions are a particular problem because they can change the chemical nature of certain DNA nucleotides (such as cytosine, designated C above) and cause mutations.

## Methane and formaldehyde

Incomplete combustion of fossil fuels, together with the evaporation of various industrial solvents, can also release a range of hydrocarbon-type substances into the atmosphere. These include acetylene, benzene, butane, propane and toluene, but by far the most abundant atmospheric hydrocarbon is *methane*, which is also released from decaying vegetation and from domestic sources. In the atmosphere, some of the methane is converted to *formaldehyde*, as a result of chemical reactions promoted by light. The ultimate concentrations in the atmosphere, however, very much depend on local climatic conditions and levels of sunlight. Indoors, formaldehyde can be slowly released from formaldehyde-based resins, or urea–formaldehyde-based insulation materials used in the building industry. Indeed, there is reason to link formaldehyde with the so-called 'sick building' syndrome that leaves occupants feeling tired, irritable and unwell, but with no specific illness. Formaldehyde can irritate the eyes, skin and throat and is believed to cause nausea, dizziness and lethargy. It may also aggravate asthma and hay fever. Although it is an established cause of skin dermatitis, there is now a worry that formaldehyde can bring about the development of cancers in experimental animals. From the chemical standpoint, this may be related to its ability to attack specific parts of DNA molecules, which can lead to the cross-linking of the individual strands of DNA molecules.

## Tobacco smoke as a pollutant

Tobacco smoke is perhaps one of the most significant atmospheric pollutants from the human health point of view, now accounting for over a third of all human cancers. It is only relatively recently that we have come to understand the dangers of tobacco. In early days, native American warriors used tobacco to make them stronger, and were convinced of its medicinal properties. Once tobacco had reached Europe, physicians also considered it to have significant medicinal properties, although many non-smokers were less convinced. However, as the dangers of smoking became more apparent in recent times, the enthusiasm amongst doctors began to wane.

By the eighteenth century, it was observed that smoking often left patients with shaking hands. Most likely this was due to nicotine withdrawal. More worrying, however, was the finding in 1761 of an English physician, John Hill, that taking snuff could lead to cancers in the nose. This still did not stop certain physicians of the time believing in the medicinal properties of tobacco, although they conceded that smoking for pleasure might not be such a good idea. Even in 1795, when Samuel Thomas von Soemmering suggested that pipe smoking could lead to lip cancer, doctors still could not agree that tobacco smoke was dangerous. Lung cancer was a rarity even in 1914: only 350 cases were reported in the whole USA. However, many more people took up smoking in World War I and rates of lung cancer incidence increased. Just at the outbreak of World War II, Franz Muller in Germany established a relationship between cancer and smoking, and the belief that smoking was health-threatening spread. On the basis of this, Hitler decreed that pilots in the Luftwaffe must not smoke so as to preserve their good health and flying skills. Despite this move, smoking in general was further accelerated by the war, and many of the vigorous advertising strategies of the tobacco companies, then and after, sought to mask any adverse medical studies. Moreover, they targeted much of their efforts on people who had not previously smoked, such as women.

Tobacco smoke is a highly complex mixture, containing over 3,500 chemicals, of which at least 40 are known to cause cancers. These include polycyclic aromatic hydrocarbons such as benzpyrene, aromatic amines and nitrosamines, which, as already mentioned, can all modify DNA nucleotide units and cause mutations. The level of such DNA modifications has been found to be higher in the DNA taken from the tissues of smokers compared with that from non-smokers. In addition to these hazardous components, the tar fraction from each puff of smoke is believed to contain as many as 100 trillion ($10^{14}$) highly reactive free radicals that can also damage DNA nucleotide units to bring about mutations.

## Atmospheric asbestos dust

Asbestos, once considered so safe that it could be used in toothpaste, is now one of the most feared contaminants on the planet. Its softness, flexibility and resistance to fire impressed initial users of asbestos.

Indeed, asbestos was once viewed as the silk of the mineral world. Over the years, people have woven asbestos cloaks, tablecloths, theatre curtains and fireproof protective clothing. Asbestos insulation products were inexpensive and useful in shielding workers from fire hazards. It was used in automobile clutch and brake manufacture as the products worked more efficiently. Asbestos was even used for domestic air filters, cigarette tips and gas masks. The irony is that the other effects of asbestos would not now loom so menacingly had it not been for its previous image as a guardian of human safety.

Asbestos dust in the atmosphere is now seen as a major human health hazard, and the use of asbestos products in the building industry is highly regulated. Building waste that is over 1 per cent contaminated with asbestos is deemed hazardous. Exposure to asbestos dust can lead to diffuse pulmonary fibrosis or cancers such as bronchiogenic cancer or malignant mesothelioma. Six main types of asbestos have been identified: actinolite, amosite, anthphyllite, crocidolite, tremolite and chrysolite. All these contain long chains of silicon and oxygen atoms that are responsible for the generally fibrous nature of the mineral, yet each type is different in its properties depending on the presence of other atoms such as iron, calcium or magnesium. The strength and resilience of asbestos make it important industrially, but it is precisely these properties that make it dangerous for human health. Asbestos fibres, particularly of the first five types, can readily penetrate our tissues, particularly in the lungs. Chrysolite, which accounts for 95 per cent of worldwide asbestos use, in relative terms may be the least hazardous, as it is notably softer than the other varieties and is more readily broken down in tissues. The potential of asbestos fibres to cause DNA damage may rest with iron atoms often found absorbed to their structure. As was suggested earlier in the case of soot particles, this absorbed iron could promote the formation of free radicals sufficiently reactive to damage DNA molecules in the vicinity of the asbestos fibres. Indeed, fibres with the highest iron content have the greatest propensity to damage DNA, and such DNA damage would serve as a source of mutations.

**Key points in this chapter**

- Since the Industrial Revolution, we have created a bizarre new chemical environment. There are now around 75,000 synthetic chemicals in common use.

- A number of synthetic chemicals are known to be capable of modifying nucleotide units of DNA. This can either be directly, or indirectly, after transformation of the chemical by proteins called cytochrome P450s.

- The various types of DNA modification include intra-strand and inter-strand cross-links. The latter type can block DNA copying and subsequent cell proliferation.

- Cytochrome P450 proteins are very diverse and there can be considerable variation between people in their response to potentially toxic chemicals.

- Two atmospheric gases whose levels are giving cause for concern are carbon dioxide and ozone. Although both contribute to the 'greenhouse' effect, ozone is also involved in the generation of smog, along with nitrogen oxides.

- Hazardous atmospheric pollutants that can modify DNA nucleotides include sulphur dioxide, formaldehyde, tobacco smoke, soot particles and asbestos dust.

# 6

# Food attack

Food is a complex affair. After sex and football there is probably no subject about which more is written and spoken. Most of us relish the pleasures of the table, and satisfy our physical requirement for nutrition at the same time. We can survive on, thrive on and enjoy a wide variety of foods. The types of foods that individuals or populations eat are influenced by many factors including availability, technology, economics, religion, cultural habits, social conditions, nutrition and taste. Although food is necessary for the support of life, for some time now we have been aware of many harmful, as well as health-giving, components associated with our diets. The impact of nutrition on chronic diseases first emerged with the discovery of vitamins in the nineteenth and twentieth centuries. Nutrition was also implicated as cancer and cardiovascular diseases began to take the place of infectious diseases as major causes of premature death in the twentieth century. As far back as 1908, in a major treatise on cancer, W.R. Williams concluded that 'the incidence of cancer is largely conditioned by nutrition'. Indeed, current knowledge on the effects of diet suggests that it is likely that, in the Western world at least, about 40 per cent of cancers may be due to diet.

Food and beverages, a large proportion of which are derived from plants, are by far the major source of chemicals entering the human body. Although we have come to expect convenience and high quality, we also want our food supply to be safe.

The problem of food safety is a very old one, but it still has many unsolved aspects. The most prevalent hazard is food-borne diseases caused by the presence of fungi or bacteria. Other food hazards include environmental contaminants, pesticide residues and additives to improve flavour and shelf life, as well as a host of natural toxins. Our food comes with a cast of extras.

## Poison on a plate

Although the manufacture in Europe of chemicals such as polychlorinated biphenyls (PCBs) was banned in the 1980s, some still occur in food. As recently as 1999 a scandal emerged in Belgium where 50 kilograms of old transformer oil containing PCBs was accidentally added to 500 tonnes of animal feed. Not surprisingly, the short-term outcome of this was a number of dead animals – in this case chickens. However, in an extensive follow-up survey, the Belgian authorities tested a vast number of food samples, including eggs, and found that around 4 per cent contained high levels of PCBs. What was worrying was the possibility that this contamination had arisen from yet another source. In the UK, the outbreak of foot and mouth disease in 2001, and the subsequent incineration of the carcasses, raised the spectre of increased dioxin levels in the atmosphere in the vicinity of the incineration sites. Dioxins are a common product of incinerated waste. During their investigations to ascertain the extent of possible dioxin fallout, the British Food Standards Agency, surprisingly, reported abnormally high levels of PCBs in eggs from a North Wales farm. Although this may be due to contaminated chicken feed, it is not possible to know for certain, as routine checks of this nature on food are not done at present. In spite of the fact that PCBs are no longer manufactured in Europe, there still remains a massive legacy in the shape of old equipment and industrial wastes.

The UK government does test several thousand food samples each year for pesticide residues. In general, the bulk of all fruit and vegetables in the UK are free of detectable pesticide residues: between a third and half do contain some, and up to 3 per cent have levels above the legal limit. Such residues mainly creep into food when the pesticides involved have been overused, or when the crops have been harvested too soon after treatment.

Pesticides are used to protect crops against damage from a wide range of pests, and because of this can increase crop yields. They are also used to minimize the damage that can occur to crops during transport and storage. They are toxic chemicals specifically employed to kill, their targets being insects, fungi and weeds, but they can also harm humans, wildlife and the environment. Occupational hazards for agricultural workers include possible long-term health problems, as well as various reproductive and neurological effects. In light of our growing knowledge of the dangers, legislation has provided some measure of safety from pesticides. However, different pesticides may be approved for use in some countries but not in others, usually because the range of crops and specific pests encountered differs from country to country. Moreover, safety evaluations usually take account of single pesticides rather than the combinations that are more usual in practice. Crops may be treated with a number of pesticides, rather than just one, over the period of their cultivation. To minimize intake of pesticide residues, it is probably good advice to wash or peel fruit and vegetables thoroughly and get rid of outer leaves. Unfortunately, although this is likely to remove surface pesticide residues, there still remains the problem of residues in the fleshy body of the fruit or vegetable. As will be discussed later in this chapter, an alternative approach to this dilemma may be to eat organically grown fruit and vegetables.

## Not all poisons are put there by man

Plants naturally manufacture an enormous range of potentially toxic compounds. Some of these are specifically to provide the plant with vital protection against infecting fungi or moulds, voracious insects and animal predators. Because plants cannot simply run away from these dangers, they have equipped themselves with the ability to turn on the manufacture of an impressive array of poisons and other noxious substances that act as natural pesticides and repellents in their fight for survival. Some of the best poisons and drugs that we know are derived from plants. These include atropine, strychnine, digitoxin, quinine, cocaine and morphine. Naturally made chemicals can be just as dangerous as synthetic chemicals. Out of the 5,000 to 10,000 natural pesticides believed to occur in the plant world, 63 have been tested so far, and, of these, 35 produced cancers in experimental rats and mice. No doubt this list will increase in the years to come. A crucial issue is one of relative dose and exposure in the test experiments with rodents. Most laboratory tests to assess toxic effects of a suspected substance are carried out over a very short time period, and with amounts of suspected toxin far in excess of what a human is likely to encounter. For instance, it has been calculated that you would have to eat 82,000 slices of bread each day for life to consume the amount of the natural substance *furfural* found to cause cancers in laboratory rats. Recall from Chapter 1 the dictum of Paracelsus that all substances are potentially poisonous; it all depends on the dose. In fact, relatively few substances that cause cancers in laboratory tests with rats and mice have actually been found to do so in humans.

It is worth pointing out that the 'natural' plant-derived pesticides have been in our diet for millions of years, which is in stark contrast to most of the synthetic pesticides presently used, which have only been with us for fifty years or much less. Many such man-made chemicals are difficult for most animals, including man, to break down within the body. As a result, there is a bodily accumulation of this type of chemical, and the higher up the food chain that an organism lives the more collects in the body. Because these chemicals enter our bodies faster than they can be eliminated, they accumulate, with the result that concentrations increase as we age. Although PCBs and dioxins are the most widely studied environmental chemicals in this respect, it is clear that our bodies now contain a veritable cocktail of chemicals that were not there fifty years ago. The reason is simple: at that time, nobody was manufacturing them.

For these sorts of reasons, many people involved at every stage of the food chain have now been persuaded to rethink their basis assumptions about the ways in which we manage the crops we grow and the food we eat. Support for *organic farming* has gathered momentum. Such practices seek to eliminate pesticides from food, and are based on the principle that, in the chain of life on earth, no species is irrelevant, and we are all interdependent from bacteria to fungi, from insects to vertebrates. Adherence to organic principles necessitates respect for the delicate relationships that exist between these species, the biosphere and humankind. It is likely that organic farming methods are a very effective way of protecting the current diversity of wildlife.

Not surprisingly, organic farming has its critics, some of whom feel that strict adherence to organic approaches is inefficient and not the ideal route to feeding an ever-growing world population. Furthermore, some approved pesticides can be used on organically grown crops, although only when there is an immediate threat to the crop. Despite this, it is clear that pesticides can drift from non-organic farms to organic ones, and in a very few cases residues of synthetic pesticides have turned up in samples of fruit and vegetables of organic origin.

Although some pesticides can undoubtedly cause various human ailments if exposure is excessive, it should be emphasized that there is insufficient evidence as yet for any direct causal link between any synthetic or natural pesticide and any human cancer (though see the section on endocrine disrupters in Chapter 11 for suspected links). In fact close inspection of possible links between cancer deaths and diet has suggested that it is the *absence* of certain components that may be more critical (see Chapter 9).

## Spoilage, preservation and cooking

The deterioration and spoilage of different types of food have often impacted on the course of history, having at times been associated with witchcraft and even miracles. An example of the latter is a bacterium called *Seratia marcescens*, dubbed the 'miracle organism', which makes a red pigment when it grows on damp foodstuffs. For this reason, it may have been responsible for the apparently miraculous 'bloodstains' on communion wafers and other breads. In general, grains, when stored under moist conditions, support the growth of various moulds. Infections of grain with one such, *Claviceps purpura*, have been well known throughout history. In the Middle Ages, epidemics of ill-health were linked to the consumption of bread and other bakery products made with contaminated rye and other grains. Such epidemics were known as St Anthony's Fire. The symptoms included inflammation of the infected tissues, followed by death of the tissues and resulting gangrene. We now know that the infecting moulds produced a group of chemicals called *ergot alkaloids*, which, in addition to being hallucinogenic, can restrict peripheral blood flow, and bring about tissue death and gangrene. Overall, many moulds are recognized for their ability to produce toxic products, which have been used by primitive tribes for religious and magical, as well as social, needs. More recent times have seen the recreational use of mind-altering agents such as *psilocybin* and *psilocin*, derived from the 'magic mushroom' *Psilocybe mexicana*. These agents were isolated and identified in 1958 by the Swiss chemist Albert Hoffman, famous for his discovery of LSD in 1943.

The contamination of foodstuffs with moulds can have a profound economic impact. Such a contamination was responsible for the outbreak of 'Turkey X' disease in the UK in the 1960s, which brought the turkey industry to its knees. Young turkeys consumed feed that was contaminated with a fungus called *Aspergillus flavus*, and developed lethargy, muscle weakness and anorexia, closely followed by spasm and death. The symptoms were brought about by toxic chemicals belonging to a group called *mycotoxins*, produced by the contaminating mould, which cause gross haemorrhaging and death of liver tissue in the afflicted turkeys.

The mycotoxins, or fungal toxins, are to be found mainly in plant-derived foods, and for this reason are likely to be of special significance to vegetarians and vegans. Moreover, current organic farming practices without the use of pesticides may further expose consumers to mycotoxins. Primarily, they are produced by fungi growing naturally in many agricultural crops, but particularly in all cereals including maize, wheat, barley, rye and oilseeds, in the field, after harvest and during storage, and later when processed into foods and animal feed concentrates. The consumption of such mycotoxin-contaminated foodstuffs can produce toxic symptoms in animals. In the field, individual animals affected by these toxins will exhibit distinctive signs of illness and in some cases will die. Acute disease symptoms can include liver failure, haemorrhaging, kidney damage, skin eruptions and tremors. Indeed, every system within the animal's body can be affected. Many toxic effects in intensively reared animals have now been ascribed to fungal mycotoxins, as the universal nature of these toxins has progressively become apparent. Unfortunately these toxins have no taste; it takes careful and costly chemical analysis to confirm their presence or otherwise. Furthermore, once present in foodstuffs they are particularly resistant to most forms of food processing, and tend to remain unchanged in the product.

At least twenty different types of mycotoxin can now be identified regularly in common agricultural crops, but especially in cereals such as maize, wheat, barley, rye and rice. Because these have different chemical structures, they can be shown to have different effects on different animal types, causing cancers, fetal deaths, birth abnormalities, dermatitis and hormone imbalances. Such effects are being reported worldwide. Fortunately, the acute forms of toxicity are not commonly seen in developed countries, since high levels of mycotoxins are less likely to occur in most commonly used agricultural products. Sadly, this is not the case in many developing countries, where warm, humid conditions and poor overall agricultural and storage management foster the growth of toxin-producing moulds. Every year, roughly 25 to 30 per cent of the world's food crops is afflicted by mycotoxins. While the serious impact on animal health and productivity is proven beyond doubt, a key question is, what is the impact on human health?

Strict food safety regulations apply in most European countries, thus minimizing the risks. Improved agricultural practices, storage and transportation systems have greatly curtailed mould growth in raw agricultural products destined for the human food chain. However, this still leaves the very real possibility of mishandling in the domestic environment (already a well recognized source of bacterial food poisoning), allowing moulds to grow and secrete toxins. At present there is still inadequate routine analysis of the human diet. Vegetarians with above-average consumption of cereals and nuts often buy these products from small suppliers, who rarely, if ever, check them for common mycotoxins. Clearly, vegetarians and vegans should be particularly vigilant, since they run a much greater risk of exposure to mycotoxins when compared to the general public. Organic farmers should also be on their guard as the lack of fungicides can open the door to mould growth, not just during crop growth but especially during prolonged periods of transport and storage. Regrettably, many practitioners of organic farming are not fully up to speed on the dangers of mycotoxins.

While food ingestion is the primary entrance route of mycotoxins for humans, another source recently implicated has been inhalation of fungal spores, particularly in contaminated damp houses. Persistent household dampness can promote fungal growth on wallpaper, plaster, and fabrics such as fitted carpets. Entry of mycotoxin fungal spores through the respiratory system is now regarded as a health risk. In animal studies the toxic potential of inhaled mycotoxins has been found to be ten times higher than that by ingestion.

## Mycotoxins and human cancer

One particular class of mycotoxin has received considerable attention, not only for its highly toxic character but also for its ability to cause cancers in a wide range of animal species, even at extremely low levels (parts per billion) in their diet. In fact these substances, the aflatoxins, are now recognized as the most potent cancer-causing substance of all naturally occurring chemicals. The fact that they occur naturally in foodstuffs for human consumption has caused much scientific and medical alarm and generated an impressive amount of research.

Critically, aflatoxins can modify DNA molecules and cause mutations. In the liver, aflatoxins are first transformed through the activities of cytochrome P450s (see Chapter 5) to a highly reactive form that has a particular affinity for joining up with nucleotides of the G-type in DNA (see Figure 6.1). One particularly potent aflatoxin, aflatoxin B1, is particularly noted for its clear association with liver cancer in humans.

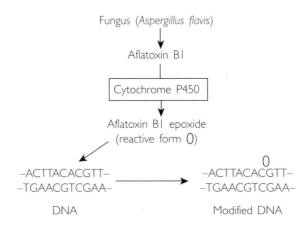

**Figure 6.1** The effect of aflatoxin B1 on DNA. Initially aflatoxin B1 is transformed by cytochrome P450 to a reactive epoxide form (represented by 0) which can then modify G-type nucleotides in DNA.

*Aspergillus* moulds that produce aflatoxin B1 are a problem because they commonly infest a wide range of commonly used foodstuffs, especially nuts and cereals. Moreover, aflatoxins have recently been detected in milk, beer, cocoa, raisins and soybean meal; as a result, governments in the Western world now severely restrict the levels of permissible contamination in these widely used foods, as well as grains and nuts. However, although products such as peanut butter are normally routinely analysed for aflatoxin by the major supermarket stores, a question remains as to whether this also happens as rigorously for products in local health food shops or farmers' markets.

## Nitrites and nitrosamines

In order to prevent food spoilage, food preservation has become an important commercial activity. Some procedures, whilst being successful in eliminating bacterial contamination, have raised further concerns regarding the potential production of novel toxic materials. For example, nitrite, a meat preservative, has been used as an antibacterial agent to retard the spore generation of a bacterium called *Clostridium botulinum*. This reduces the rate of spoilage and also protects the consumer against botulism. The nitrite, in small amounts, is also responsible for the reddening effect and the preservation of flavour in cured meats. Despite these desirable effects, nitrite is also the culprit in the formation of nitrosamines from the amines and amino acids in certain cured meats, such as bacon, under the high temperatures of pan-frying. These nitrosamines are known to be capable of causing mutations, which could be the result of an ability to link up with nucleotides in DNA. However, so far, solid evidence linking such nitrosamines with any human cancer is lacking.

In the 1980s there was a scare that nitrates in food, stemming from the overenthusiastic use of fertilizers, could be acted upon by bacteria in the mouth and saliva to produce nitrites. In turn, these nitrites were believed to react in the stomach with products of digestion to yield nitrosamines that could possibly cause stomach or oesophageal cancer. Around that time clinicians had noted a sinister increase in the occurrence of cancers, particularly around the gastro-oesophageal junction, where the oesophagus joins the stomach. This increase followed the same pattern as the increase in use of nitrate fertilizer, but with a ten- to twenty-year time lag. As we shall see in later chapters, this time lag is a familiar feature of environmental cancer development. Twenty years ago, the condition afflicted 450 Scots each year, some as young as in their thirties, but now the figure is nearer 900, and gastro-oesophageal cancer is Scotland's most rapidly increasing cancer. Unfortunately, a healthy lifestyle may not help. We get 80 per cent of our nitrates from fruit and vegetables; worse still, washing your lettuce or boiling your potatoes does not remove these nitrates. Even organic produce may not be the answer, as the manures often used may still contain nitrates. There is certainly an urgent case for further research to establish whether such food-borne nitrates are truly the causative agents. It is already clear that this cancer afflicts some people and not others, and research specifically involving workers at a factory manufacturing ammonium nitrate fertilizer, and thus well exposed to nitrates, has so far drawn a blank. Whatever their basis, these scares may well have contributed to the present reduction in the use of nitrite as a meat preservative.

## Irradiation of food

Other approaches to food preservation have involved the use of radiation such as ultraviolet type C (UVC) and gamma rays. UVC radiation (see Chapter 8) is lethal to bacteria, but, unfortunately, does not penetrate glass and water very effectively. In the main, UVC is used in rather restricted situations such as the sterilization of air systems or working surfaces. For the sterilization of water, equipment is required that allows only thin layers of water to pass under strong UV lamps.

Unlike UVC, ionizing radiation in the shape of gamma rays (see Chapter 3) can penetrate through glass and water and deep into objects. In principle, ionizing radiation can be used to control insect and microbial infestations of food and thereby reduce the dangers from food-poisoning bacteria. In recent years, there has been considerable concern caused by the apparent increases in human illnesses caused by foods contaminated by poisonous bacteria. Most of us have experienced food poisoning in its most familiar form of distressing episodes of diarrhoea and/or vomiting, fortunately usually of relatively short duration. Few of us will now be unaware of the food poisoning potential of bacteria such as *Salmonella* and *E. coli* 0157:H7. The latter type is particularly unpleasant as it produces toxic substances that cause bloody diarrhoea, and sometimes kidney failure and death.

At present, gamma radiation from a cobalt 60 source is routinely used for the cold sterilization of antibiotics, sutures and disposable plastic items, such as syringes, for clinical use. The use of nuclear radiation for food preservation has not gained universal public acceptance, although it is actually permitted for certain specified foods in more than thirty countries, where it has been used to treat poultry and extend the shelf life of seafoods and fruits. (It became legal in the UK in 1991.) Perhaps understandably, there is public hostility to the use of a type of radiation that has such a chequered history in relation to our health and well-being (see Chapter 3). In the case of food irradiation, some of this public apprehension is misplaced. Nuclear radiation produces very few chemical changes in food, in reality far less than produced for example by cooking. In general the losses of vitamins from food exposed to the low doses of radiation normally used are much less than in cooking. So far, the best results have been with meat, fish, eggs, seeds and herbs. Because the main constituent of most food is water, the major products arising from irradiation, as will be appreciated from Chapter 3, are free radicals from that water. These radicals are highly reactive and can, of course, be seriously damaging if produced in close proximity to biologically important molecules such as the DNA of any bacteria contaminating the food. Contaminating bacteria will be killed, but what is also beneficial is that, after irradiation of the food, these free radicals disappear spontaneously and virtually instantaneously. Crucially, they thus present no danger to consumers eating the food many days or weeks later. On the other hand, some free radicals, produced in rigid food structures such as bone or cellulose of irradiated fish and chicken, and also some fruits, persist long enough to be ingested. Some of these vanish rapidly when exposed to moisture, and there is no evidence that any of these particular types of free radical constitute a hazard to health. Irradiation, as a method of eliminating bacterial contaminations, because it is so efficient and uses relatively low doses of nuclear radiation, is likely to be more extensively utilized in the future. Astronauts already eat irradiated food, as do people with weakened immune systems. Hopefully, these uses will help to reduce growing public hysteria over food safety issues, and assist a harassed food industry searching for some way of cleaning up its act after so many recent food-poisoning incidents involving bacteria such as *Salmonella* and *E. coli* 0157:H7.

## Cooking

When food is cooked, burnt material is often produced, some components of which can lead to cancers, as observed in experimental animals. Roasted coffee contains some 1,000 different chemicals; of 28 so far tested, 19 cause cancers in experimental animals. On the face of it, this sort of evidence seems quite alarming. Our diets would seem to be a prime source of compounds potentially hazardous to DNA. In the case of coffee, however, there is absolutely no evidence to indicate that drinking it in the normal amounts is a cancer risk for humans. This somewhat paradoxical situation again highlights an important issue already touched on. The high concentrations of these apparently harmful dietary components that have to administered to experimental animals to cause cancers bear little significant relationship to the very much lower concentrations consumed by humans on a daily basis. This is a consideration that must temper all our views of the potential hazards of food.

During the last ten years or so, a group of chemicals called *heterocyclic amines* have been isolated from fried, broiled, deep-fried or baked meat and fish. Similar chemical substances can also be created in the laboratory if mixtures of creatinine, amino acids and sugars are heated to temperatures of between 125 and 200 degrees Celsius. Significantly, creatinine, amino acids and sugars all occur naturally in the muscles of fish and animal meat. We now know that more than a dozen heterocyclic amines appear to be capable of producing mutations in DNA and some can even form links with DNA. For these reasons, heterocyclic amines may also be potentially hazardous for us, although once more it should be emphasized that no studies as yet indicate any clear links with human cancers.

## New genes on the menu

Perhaps the biggest changes likely to affect the food we eat in the future will be the result of genetic engineering. Most people in the UK have already eaten food produced using this technique, and the same is probably true of many other industrialized countries. Crops such as soybean and maize have been genetically engineered and products from them have been mixed with those from unmodified varieties for transport and marketing. Effectively this has made them physically inseparable, and so a considerable range of food potentially contains genetically engineered ingredients.

For over 10,000 years we have cultivated plants and, by selective breeding techniques, have made continuous improvements to these to meet our varying food requirements. However, the new techniques of genetic engineering differ from these traditional methods in fundamental ways. Although plant breeding will continue to be available to provide crop improvements, it will always be limited by the sexual compatibility of the plants concerned. Because of this, cross-fertilization between different species cannot occur. That puts a limit on the number of genes available for the improvement of a particular plant species. Genetic engineering, by breaking down such barriers, opens up new possibilities, creating new genetic combinations for the breeders. Genetic engineering provides a means whereby genes can cross the barriers between species. This is because the transfer of genes can now be achieved in ways that are not possible in the natural world. Furthermore, once a gene from one species has been engineered into another, it can be passed on, like any other gene to its progeny, using the traditional methods.

In 1985, the first foreign gene was transferred into a plant, in this case tobacco. In the next ten years, over sixty other plants were genetically engineered and roughly 3,000 field tests involving such plants carried out worldwide. Most of these early efforts were aimed at producing plants with increased resistance to specific herbicides. It was envisaged that this would permit more efficient control of weeds, as the weed-killing herbicides used would be less able to damage the crops. As yet, crop plants are the main group of genetically engineered organism to enter our food chain, and this predominantly as ingredi-

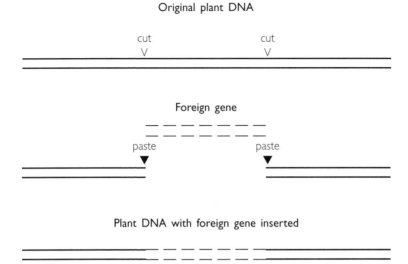

**Figure 6.2** A schematic illustration of the basic elements of genetic engineering in which a foreign gene is inserted into the DNA of an organism (such as a plant), by a process analogous to 'cutting and pasting'.

ents of processed foods. Other products include tomatoes modified for longer shelf life.

How does genetic engineering work? It seeks, by the manipulation of genes in the test tube, to introduce, enhance or delete particular characteristics of an organism such as a plant. You will recall from Chapter 2 that a gene is basically a segment of DNA that carries the code for making a particular protein. Think of genes as a strip of audiotape. Then imagine this strip being cut in places with scissors, and the pieces reassembled in a different order with some sort of glue, a sort of 'cut and paste' job. Now the audiotape will include a 'tune' spliced in from a different tape. Molecular biologists use a group of proteins, called *restriction enzymes*, which act as 'scissors' to cut DNA where they want. In this way, they can chop out a gene from the DNA of one organism and then put it into another (Figure 6.2). In short, it is possible to transplant a gene; if done correctly, the recipient organism will have a new working gene. It will now do something different, because it will be instructed to make a new type of protein. It will be a changed creature and, furthermore, will pass its changed character to its offspring. If you let the new organism multiply, you have cloned the organism. A *clone* is essentially a genetic copy. An organism that contains strips of 'foreign' DNA is called a *recombinant organism.*

This revolutionary technique of genetic engineering began in 1973 when Stanley Cohen and Herbert Boyer, along with others, succeeded in putting working foreign genes into bacteria called *Escherichia coli* that normally live in the human gut (this variety is not to be confused with the dangerous *Escherichia coli* 0157:H7, mentioned previously). Because of these foreign genes, which they now contained, the bacteria took on different characteristics. Cohen and Boyer shared the Nobel Prize for this historic experiment in twentieth-century science. The genes they transplanted gave *Escherichia coli* resistance to certain antibiotics. The organisms, with their new properties, however, were not dangerous and were readily wiped out by other antibiotics. The experiment was completely safe. These biotechnological achievements led to the growth of a new set of industries, particularly in the USA, the UK and Japan.

Despite claims for the apparent safety of the technique, many scientists very soon became worried that moving genes from one bacterium to another could cause outbreaks of new infectious diseases, or even environmental disasters. Concerned scientists urged a temporary halt in genetic experimentation until the scientific community could debate the hazards and produce some sort of guidelines to ensure safe working practices and prevent accidents. A large meeting to debate these issues was held in Asilomar, California, in 1975. The Asilomar Conference, as it became known, brought a sense of reason to a situation that had initially seemed somewhat frightening. After the conference, scientists proceeded with considerable caution. A set of guidelines, the Asilomar Safety Guidelines, was established for carrying out genetic engineering experiments, and a number of safety review boards and procedures were put in place.

While guidelines exist to facilitate safe progress, there are still a number of questions that clearly trouble the public at large – and, indeed, some scientists. In the particular context of food, it still is very much a battle for hearts and minds. Many big multinational companies sincerely believed that the application of genetic engineering in the food industry would be greeted with enthusiasm in the market place. They took the view that there would be many beneficial effects for crop production and the environment. It was thus quite a shock for them to find that a significant proportion of the public felt that the food-related products of genetic engineering were 'contaminated' in some way. Undoubtedly there is also public concern over the moral acceptability of genetic engineering. This will have to be faced squarely before any further commercial development is possible. Even Charles, Prince of Wales, has allegedly asked whether we have the right to experiment with, and commercialize, the building blocks of life.

A simple basic question is whether food containing genetically engineered products is safe to eat. Are there problems when it comes to eating genes, particularly alien ones? We eat the genes of many animals and plants in our everyday diet, cooked or otherwise. We have always done this, with apparently no ill effect. However, due to the particular nature of genetically engineered foods, inasmuch as genes are transplanted between different species during their production, the possibility of unpredictable outcomes should not be discounted. For instance, because a particular plant product might contain a novel protein arising from a gene transplanted to that plant from another species, it may well cause allergic reactions in some consumers that were not foreseen. Already 1 to 2 per cent of the populations of most Western countries have an allergic reaction to one food type or another. Evaluation of the possible allergic properties of engineered plant products is possible. Although present testing takes account of this issue, it may not be possible, at this stage, for the analyses used to be completely exhaustive. Another concern arises from the present inability of the new technology to transplant genes to precise locations in the recipient plant chromosomes. Because an incoming gene is essentially parachuted in, its landing spot might well be in the middle, or close to, plant genes for making the toxic compound that normally protects it from predators. Thus, it is not impossible that this untargeted gene transfer might affect the way in which the recipient plant is programmed to make these natural toxins. If produced by the plant in larger than normal amounts, these could present health dangers for humans if they become incorporated in food products. It is not impossible to test engineered plants for toxins that are either unusual, or occur at concentrations higher than normal. As far as can be discerned, no such testing is envisaged by any commercial or government body.

Yet another worry is that bacteria which live normally in our intestines might acquire resistance to certain antibiotics from so-called marker genes in engineered plants. Marker genes are normally inserted into engineered plants simply to identify those plants that have been engineered from those that have not. The genes used to provide this tagging function are usually bacterial genes that encode resistance to certain antibiotics. Microorganisms routinely produce antibiotics as a defence against predatory bacteria, but, over time, these bacteria often develop resistance to the damaging effects of antibiotics. The genes in such bacteria, which direct the manufacture of proteins that make them resistant, can be isolated and transferred to plants. Popular marker genes are those from bacteria that encode resistance to kanamycin, neomycin and ampicillin. The idea is to locate these tags close to the genes for the desired characteristic to be transferred to the recipient plant. Thus, if the desired genes have been successfully transplanted, so also will be the marker gene. In this way, not only will the resultant plant have the new desired characteristics, but also it can be readily distinguished from others by virtue of its newly acquired antibiotic resistance.

A snag in this scenario, as perceived by many critics, is that many of the antibiotics used to distinguish the engineered plants are in common clinical and veterinary use in many countries, although studies claim that antibiotic resistance genes pose no threat to humans. The issue hinges around the possibility that the antibiotic resistance genes will be transferred to the bacteria normally living in our intestines, or those of agricultural animals. As we shall see in the next chapter, it is true that genes can be transferred naturally to bacteria and so the possibility is not unrealistic. However, it has to be realized that our digestive systems act as a natural barrier against DNA. The acidic conditions in the gut of animals and humans break down most DNA. Nevertheless, there have been studies where some DNA, fed orally to mice, has survived in the gut, and so the possibility of gene transfer cannot be completely ruled out. If it were to occur, then the clinical or veterinary use of certain antibiotics would become less effective. The risks would be much reduced in the case of cooked foods or highly processed products where any DNA would be destroyed. In any event, to pre-empt these risks, there have been moves towards the use of different types of marker genes, and more appropriate ones may soon emerge. For the moment, just as there are genuine scientific concerns regarding the safety of organic farming products, the same is true of products based on the use of genetically engineered plants.

---

**Key points in this chapter**

- Despite bans on their manufacture and use, residues of synthetic chemicals such as PCBs still contaminate our food.
- Despite legislation to minimize their use, synthetic pesticides also contaminate some food products, albeit at a comparatively low level.
- There are as yet no direct links between any synthetic or natural pesticides and DNA damage or cancer in humans.
- Fungal infection of foodstuffs can be hazardous by virtue of myco-toxin production. This could be a problem for organic farmers.
- One particular mycotoxin, aflatoxin B1, can be transformed in cells to a form that is able to modify certain DNA components. It has been specifically associated with human stomach cancers.
- Nitrites are used as food preservatives, and, under some conditions, can give rise to nitrosamines that can damage DNA. However, at the levels normally encountered, they are not a known health risk, and no specific evidence links them with human cancers.
- Food preservation with ionizing radiation is likely to be very useful. Although free radicals are formed in the irradiated food, these are short lived and present no dangers for the consumer.
- Cooking of some foods can also produce substances that can cause cancers in animals, but no studies so far link any of these with human cancers.

- Food products made from plants that have been genetically engineered might cause allergic reactions in some consumers. Genetically engineered plants could also contain more than the normal levels of natural toxins, which could be hazardous if incorporated into food. Transfer of bacterial marker genes in the plant products to bacteria in the human intestine might prejudice the future clinical use of some antibiotics, but choice of different genetic markers could alleviate such problems.

# Enemies from within

You might get the impression from all that has been said so far that, if you avoided exposure to sunlight, nuclear radiation, tobacco smoke, car exhaust fumes, asbestos, mycotoxins, toxic chemicals and other industrial pollutants, your DNA would remain unharmed. Unfortunately, it is not so. As time goes by, your DNA would still become damaged. When examined closely, a considerable proportion of the damage to DNA is indicative of the work of free radicals.

## What are free radicals?

Free radicals are chemical entities that, characteristically, have an unpaired electron in their make-up. They cause a problem because they can 'mug' a variety of molecules in cells, with the general aim of stealing a precious electron to re-establish the normal pairing of their own electrons. If the mugging is successful, the victim molecule is left with a deficiency of electrons, which can lead to knock-on problems such as structural disintegration. Although it requires very sophisticated analytical equipment to detect free radicals themselves, it is relatively easy to spot the chemical footprints they leave behind, because they damage DNA in a characteristic way. You may recall from Chapter 3 that free radicals are generated from the water of cells and tissues when exposed to ionizing radiation. Even in the absence of such radiation, it is now evident that similar, damaging free radicals are generated normally as we fight infections and as we turn food into energy. Despite the fact that these processes are necessary for life and health, the free radicals generated are nonetheless potentially hazardous. They can contribute directly, and indirectly, to a low level of unwelcome damage to cell molecules, including DNA.

## Free radicals fight infection

*Neutrophils* and *macrophages* are specialized cells of the immune system that patrol in the bloodstream, seeking out any invading infectious organisms such as bacteria and viruses. Should such organisms be encountered, these special cells quickly engulf them. Once inside, the foreign organisms are efficiently killed using a mechanism that involves free radicals generated from oxygen. One important type produced is *superoxide radicals*. Although not very toxic themselves, superoxide radicals can readily give rise to *hydrogen peroxide*, which is highly damaging to bacteria and viruses. Furthermore, hydrogen peroxide can give rise to extremely reactive *hydroxyl radicals*.

The initial generation of superoxide radicals is thus central to the overall killing process, which is a fundamental component of immunological protection, ensuring that invading infectious organisms are eliminated from our bodies. Patients with chronic granulomatous disease are unable to generate these vital superoxide radicals. This makes it difficult for them to defend themselves against invading organisms, and they are vulnerable to persistent multiple infections of the skin, lungs, liver and bone.

Despite its vital role, this bodily defence mechanism involving free radicals is not without its hazards. As already mentioned, superoxide radicals can spontaneously give rise to hydrogen peroxide. This product can be problematic, as it is a potential source of damaging hydroxyl radicals. If hydrogen peroxide comes in contact with any free iron atoms within cells, hydroxyl radicals can result. The difficulty is that these radicals can diffuse from the sites of their creation and cause damage to fats and DNA within innocent healthy tissues and cells that just happen to be close by. This is a significant cost to be set against the general benefits of the lifelong battles against infection mounted by the immune system. Conditions of chronic inflammation such as inflammatory bowel disease and rheumatoid arthritis are notable for the intensity of free radical generation as neutrophils and macrophages cluster at sites of inflammation. In the case of the inflamed rheumatoid knee joint, a flux of free radicals, propagated from immune cells, is likely to contribute significantly to the structural damage suffered by molecules in the tissues and cells of the joint. Examination of the synovial fluid from the knee joints of patients has revealed the characteristic footprints of free radicals. In the light of this finding, various possible therapeutic approaches are being evaluated. These involve the use either of drugs that can generally mop up free radicals, or of others that can specifically remove iron atoms from the vicinity of the inflammation, thus diminishing the opportunity for the formation of the highly damaging hydroxyl radicals from hydrogen peroxide.

In addition to the natural production of free radicals in the defence against infection, there is yet another source within the body where free radicals are naturally produced.

## Free radicals arise from energy production

Surprisingly perhaps, the oxygen in air is potentially dangerous. How can this be? Surely oxygen molecules from the atmosphere are fundamentally important for sustaining life? The danger arises from the fact that oxygen picks up electrons in a chain of complex sequential biochemical reactions that occur in cells for the production of energy from food. These particular reactions are orchestrated within special structures lying inside all cells called *mitochondria* (see Figure 2.4). Unfortunately, due to what might be thought of as accidents of their chemistry, certain components of these mitochondria can inappropriately leak electrons directly to oxygen. Because oxygen has the capacity to accept one electron at a time, superoxide radicals can result. Although these superoxide radicals tend to remain within mitochondria, they can spontaneously change into hydrogen peroxide molecules, which, unlike superoxide radicals, can diffuse from the mitochondria and become distributed throughout the rest of the cell. As will be recalled, hydrogen peroxide can be a very real problem within cells, as it is a potential source of damaging hydroxyl radicals.

Recent estimates indicate that as much as 2 to 5 per cent of the oxygen consumed by mitochondria may be inappropriately converted to superoxide radicals, a first step in the production of hydroxyl radicals.

In short, the very utilization of food for the creation of the energy necessary for everyday activities inconveniently begets yet another significant risk for the DNA of our genes. Together with the damaging free radicals continuously emerging from the immune defence systems, the free radicals originating from mitochondria constitute a significant threat to DNA, but it is a threat that emerges from within our cells rather than from any external environmental source.

## How damaging is the free radical assault on DNA?

The extent of damage to DNA from such apparently 'natural' internal sources is surprisingly high. At any one time, it is estimated that around 150,000 nucleotides are found to be damaged by this route out of the total of 3 billion nucleotides that constitute the DNA molecules found in each cell. Surprisingly, this is about ten- to a hundredfold more than the number of nucleotides likely to be found damaged as a result of our exposure to the range of external environmental sources that we normally encounter at the present time. When the level of damage due to attack by internally generated free radicals is compared among different species, it appears to be related to the rate at which the mitochondria create energy in different species. For example, the DNA of rodents, whose mitochondria operate at a higher rate than those of humans, seems to show more damage than the DNA of humans. This again generally supports the view that a flux of DNA-damaging free radicals arises from the mitochondria where the energy conversion processes take place. Moreover, the extent of this naturally caused damage accumulates with the age of the animal. In aged animals, the level of such damage is around twice that found in young animals.

In short, the process of internal attack from free radicals is likely to be a major contributor to the significant damage that our DNA accumulates over a lifetime. In turn, this has served as the basis for arguments that free radical damage to DNA is a major component of the ageing processes; we shall return to this aspect in Chapter 10. It is the price we have to pay for living in an atmosphere containing oxygen and using free radicals to stave off bacterial and viral infections.

## The natural instability of our DNA

For some time after its discovery, it was, quite reasonably, believed that DNA was stable, and, except for a few random mutations, that it passed unchanged from generation to generation. This view has had to change. Research in recent years has shown that DNA is a much more dynamic molecule than initially suspected.

### Spontaneous decay

In addition to the age-related degeneration of DNA due to continuous bombardment by free radicals, as just outlined, there are chemical features of DNA itself that contribute to its *spontaneous degeneration.* Even under the normal physiological conditions that prevail within cells, certain parts of the nucleotide units that make up DNA can alter spontaneously. This is simply a feature of their chemical construction. It is almost as if they have a built-in shelf life. The level of such spontaneous alterations is surprisingly high. Indeed, a figure of 10,000 spontaneously altered nucleotides in every cell generation has been suggested. In principle, alteration of DNA nucleotide units on this scale could cause considerable gene damage. During the ensuing DNA replication processes, the copying machinery would not be able to place the correct nucleotides in response to the altered nucleotide units on the DNA strands being copied. However, as will be seen in Chapter 9, repair systems exist within cells to remove most of these altered nucleotides, and thereby minimize the extent of such spontaneous gene damage.

### Problems when copying DNA

Although the machinery that copies DNA works with almost perfect fidelity, there are nevertheless a few mistakes made. Fortunately, the majority of these errors are corrected by a team of 'proof-reading' proteins that check the copies every few steps. Where errors are detected, these are 'snipped out' and the DNA replaced correctly at that spot. Sometimes the copying apparatus can have difficulties at places in DNA where the sequence of DNA nucleotides repeats itself. For example, there may be a stretch containing the sequence –CACACACA–, and, as if the copying machinery becomes a little confused, the new strand produced at this location can have too many, or too few, nucleotides – for example, –GTGTGTGTGTG– or –GTGTGT–. The official name for this type of copying fault is *replication slippage*. There can also be situations when the DNA strands to be copied become misaligned, leading to an extra nucleotide, or nucleotides, being inserted in the copy produced. Conversely, too few nucleotides in the copy are also a possibility in this type of situation. Such errors have obvious consequences when the affected region of DNA is decoded. Essentially, they are a form of mutation.

## DNA that jumps

Recent research has suggested that as much as a third of our DNA consists of segments that could move, or that have moved sometime in our evolutionary past. Fortunately, we have chemical mechanisms for keeping this mobile DNA in check. Clearly there could be significant problems if chunks of such DNA could regularly 'up sticks' and insert themselves elsewhere, possibly in some vital gene. However, in some species this does sometimes happen and the proper decoding of the DNA at the site of insertion can be afflicted.

In the 1940s, Barbara McClintock at the Cold Spring Harbor Laboratory, New York, was the first person to advance the idea of DNA that could jump from one site on one chromosome to another. During classic experiments on maize, she characterized genetic entities that could move into (as well as out of) genes, thus changing the attributes of the maize kernels. At the time her views were treated with extreme scepticism. However, by the 1970s mobile DNA elements in bacteria, now called *transposons*, had been discovered. These are extremely common in bacteria, where they can copy themselves and can insert the copies at any point in bacterial DNA, and often cause serious disruption to the function of genes so targeted. They are also common in plants, where they are referred to as *transposable elements*. Maize has several varieties of transposable elements, which act to move genes around chromosomes. Such elements can range from a few hundred nucleotides in length to a few thousand nucleotides, and the process whereby these segments of DNA are copied and inserted at new sites is called *transposition*. Mobile DNA elements are essentially parasites that appear, as far as we know, to have no specific function in the biology of the organism harbouring them. They seem to exist only to maintain themselves. For this reason Francis Crick called them selfish DNA. This does not mean that they carry genes for making organisms selfish. Rather, it merely describes their particular lifestyle. Although environmental influences on their behaviour cannot be ruled out, equally there is no evidence to support such a possibility.

Since McClintock's pioneering studies, transposable elements have been identified in insects. Other animals, including humans, also appear to have DNA sequences that have some similarities with transposable elements. Although their present significance is not clear, there is speculation that they may have played some genetic role in our evolutionary past. Over the millions of years of evolutionary time, the transposition of mobile elements is believed to have resulted in their accumulation in human DNA. Because they are eliminated only very slowly, they have built up to a point such that they now constitute a significant proportion of our total DNA. Whether or not these processes have been influenced by environmental factors during evolutionary time must remain a speculation for the present.

## Insertion of genes into human DNA

The discovery of sequences in DNA with the some of the characteristics of mobile DNA has certainly transformed views of the human genome. It now seems more plastic and amenable to experimentation than had previously been imagined. If segments of DNA can move, the question arises, could we purposely insert DNA segments of our own design into human chromosomes? Clearly we would first have to understand the rules that govern such processes, but this would be a possible route to inserting specific DNA segments as a means of correcting or replacing defective human genes. This would be an example of a mutation that could be positively beneficial.

As will be more fully considered in Chapter 14, various means of attempting to cure human disease by this route have been considered. The crucial question is, how can the correct DNA be inserted into the correct chromosomes? A group of viruses that can infect cells, the *retroviruses*, seem almost to be standing by to provide an answer to this question. These viruses have an extremely complex reproductive cycle.

A particularly well-known example is the human immunodeficiency virus, or *HIV* for short. Readers will probably be familiar with this virus in relation to the development of acquired immunodeficiency syndrome, or *AIDS*. Virologists working in France and the United States first identified this virus in 1983 as the causative agent. In the case of AIDS, the critical target of the virus is a group of T-cells that are part of the white blood cell population central to the functioning of the immune system. The HIV virus can readily enter human cells, hijack their machinery and make more copies of themselves. Although the genes of this, and other retroviruses, are actually made of RNA rather than DNA, during the infectious process this RNA is converted to a DNA equivalent which is inserted into the DNA of the infected cell's nucleus. Thus, a copy of the retrovirus in terms of DNA is left behind in the chromosomes of the infected cell. The site of integration of this DNA equivalent, however, appears to be random. This can have potentially harmful consequences for the subsequent life of the infected cell. For example, crucial genes might be interrupted and the behaviour of that cell, and its descendants, permanently afflicted. Curiously, many segments of our DNA that have the outward appearance of transposable elements, as described above, in fact have many characteristics similar to those of DNA segments inserted during retrovirus infection. Their precise origin in evolutionary time remains uncertain, however. Despite having no apparent direct function, other than the maintenance of their own existence, their presence nonetheless may have had a profound effect, at some time, on the evolution of modern mankind. They may conceivably have led to the evolution of new genes, or new controls of gene activity. The view that they are simply selfish parasites may well turn out to be premature.

While our increasing knowledge of retroviruses, such as HIV, may help us find a solution to the AIDS problem, it may well also assist us to find less hazardous retroviruses to use as Trojan Horses for transporting and inserting DNA into cells to replace defective genes that occur in heritable diseases such as cystic fibrosis. However, there will be more on that subject later (see Chapter 14).

**Key points in this chapter**

- Free radicals are generated naturally in the fight against infection and during the chemical processes involved in obtaining energy from food.
- These internally generated free radicals cause a surprisingly high level of damage to DNA, equivalent to ten to a hundred times that caused by exposure to the normally encountered level of environmental agents.
- DNA itself is inherently unstable. Some nucleotide units show a slow rate of spontaneous alteration.
- The DNA copying machinery of cells can occasionally make mistakes, although proof-reading mechanisms exist.
- Transposable elements and transposons are DNA segments found in a variety of organisms that can move from one DNA location to another. They may have played a role in our evolution.
- DNA can also be inserted into chromosomes from external sources such as retroviruses.

# 8

# A first line of defence

In 1985, the British Antarctic Atmospheric Survey rang alarm bells around the world when they discovered that ozone levels in the stratosphere (10–40 km above sea level) over the South Pole were dwindling alarmingly during the months of September and October, the time when the sun returns at the end of the polar spring. Worse still, this thinning had been going on since the 1960s. By 1987, Antarctic ozone levels, over an area corresponding to the size of the USA, were around half that of normal.

Why all the fuss? Up until about 3 billion years ago there was no oxygen whatsoever in the earth's atmosphere. Around that time, in a period referred to by geologists as the Precambrian, a group of bacteria, the *cyanobacteria*, evolved the ability to carry out the complex biochemical processes that we now called photosynthesis. Broadly speaking, these involve the capture of light energy and its conversion to chemical energy stored in the form of sugars and other molecules, which are subsequently used by the bacteria for their survival and reproduction. From this period on, life on earth became progressively more solar-powered. Oxygen is a notable waste product of photosynthesis, and over the next few billion years the concentration of oxygen rose to as much as 35 per cent. This high level was due to the fact that there were no life forms that used oxygen at that time. Gradually, however, organisms that could use oxygen did evolve and the atmospheric oxygen concentration fell to its present level of 21 per cent. It was the high atmospheric levels of oxygen that led to the formation of ozone. Up in the stratosphere, oxygen molecules absorb high-energy radiation from the sun and some break up to give free radicals that can interact with some of the remaining oxygen to yield ozone. The crucial effects of this ozone layer are now beginning to be fully appreciated. It is a first line of defence, serving to filter out the most harmful types of solar radiation and thereby shielding us from its worst effects.

## The role of the ozone layer

Not all types of potentially harmful solar radiation can penetrate the entire atmosphere and reach the earth's surface. Solar X-rays, gamma rays, infrared radiation and most cosmic rays are screened out. Fortunately, the short-wavelength ultraviolet rays of a type called *UVC*, which could cause very severe damage to DNA, are also completely filtered out by the atmosphere. Only certain radio waves and radiation around the wavelength of visible light, together with some short-wavelength infrared, and longer-wavelength ultraviolet rays, called *UVA* and *UVB*, can reach sea level to bombard exposed skin and eyes. Although UVA rays are not normally associated with direct damage to DNA, they can cause indirect effects such as tanning or inflammation to skin tissue. In contrast, UVB rays can cause severe sunburn and cataracts of the eye as well as being able to damage DNA and bring about the development of skin cancers. Providentially, the accumulation of a layer of ozone molecules provides a barrier to UVB penetration.

**Table 8.1**    Ultraviolet radiation from the sun

| Type | Wavelength (nm) | Effect |
| --- | --- | --- |
| UVA | 315–400 | Causes skin tanning and tissue inflammation; passes through the ozone layer. |
| UVB | 280–315 | Causes sunburn, cataracts, damage to DNA and skin cancers; ozone layer screens out 99 per cent. |
| UVC | < 280 | Can severely damage DNA; completely screened out by the ozone layer. |

This ozone layer is normally 99 per cent effective in screening out hazardous UVB radiation (see Table 8.1).

There was no cause for concern until the alarming observations of the British Antarctic Atmospheric Survey in 1985. In 1995–96, a loss of ozone of around 10 per cent was reported from the stratosphere in the region of the North Pole. This came on top of considerable losses over the previous few winters. However, these particular winters were unusual in that the Arctic stratosphere had stayed colder for longer than usual. Some observers have suggested that global warming may also make a contribution to these effects. While climatic change is warming the atmosphere closer to the ground, it is cooling the lower stratosphere. Despite the lack of a clear understanding, many scientists believe that colder temperatures in the stratosphere may worsen the depletion of ozone.

## Why is the ozone layer thinning?

The depletion of ozone from the stratosphere has certainly stirred up much fervent debate, as it is likely to have serious consequences for life on earth. For instance, for every 5 per cent depletion in stratospheric ozone, it is estimated that there would be a 10 per cent increase in UVB penetration to sea level. Apart from the losses at the poles, there has been a global loss of stratospheric ozone over the last two decades of around 8 per cent. Although plants are relatively resistant to UV damage, having quite efficient screening mechanisms, humans can look forward to increased skin ageing and cancers unless we can minimize the extent of our exposure.

How has this come about? There are two current hypotheses to explain the changes in polar ozone. One suggests that the cause could simply be the breakdown, at springtime, in the southern hemisphere, of the complex polar wind systems. The other, perhaps more sinister and the recipient of intense publicity, is founded on the possibility that, in a set of complex chemical reactions, chlorofluorocarbons (CFCs) in the atmosphere are broken down by light, or in reactions with oxygen, to yield chlorine. In turn, the chlorine can destroy many ozone atoms by forming chlorine oxides.

## Chlorofluorocarbons

Thomas Midgley invented the first of the chlorofluorocarbons, namely *Freon*, around 1930. He has already featured in this book. In 1921 he found that lead in petrol would improve the performance of automobile engines (see Chapter 5). His efforts made high-compression engines for both automobiles and aeroplanes a possibility. Following these successes, the General Motors Fridgidaire Division persuaded Midgley to take on the problems of refrigeration, with the resultant invention of Freon. Apparently he demonstrated the properties of his invention to the assembled members of the American Chemical Society by inhaling a lungful and then exhaling in the direction of a lit candle that was duly extinguished as a result. Lead in petrol and Freon were not his only achievements; he held an impressive number of other patents and was the recipient of many prestigious awards in the USA for his contributions to the advancement of chemistry. He was a highly ingenious inventor; even when he was struck down with polio in 1940, he devised a complex arrangement of pulleys and cords to assist him in and out of bed. However, a cruel stroke of irony contributed to his death in 1944. He was accidentally strangled as a result of becoming enmeshed in the network of ropes and pulleys that he had invented for himself. A stroke of monstrous bad luck perhaps, but a fitting epitaph might be an observation from the historian John McNeill that Midgley has had more impact on our atmosphere than any other single organism.

It was only after World War II that Midgley's CFCs really caught on. Among other things, CFCs turned out to be extremely effective as solvents and as components of refrigerants and spray propellants. They were particularly useful in these roles because of their lack of toxicity and non-flammable nature. CFCs were also seen as safe because they reacted with hardly anything. However, there was a problem once they rose to the higher reaches of the atmosphere, where they did react in the presence of solar radiation to release chlorine, which in turn ruptured ozone molecules. Up until the end of the Second World War, CFC releases into the atmosphere were relatively small. However, by the 1970s, emissions were such that the integrity of the ozone layer was at risk. Some scientists had already suggested that thinning of the ozone layer was more than just a theoretical possibility. A sobering thought is that a single CFC molecule released at ground level can take around fifteen years to reach the stratosphere. Even the chlorine produced as a result of CFC degradation remains in the stratosphere for some considerable time. Moreover, each chlorine molecule can destroy many thousands of stratospheric ozone molecules.

Inadvertently, modifying the earth's stratosphere through the manufacture and release of CFCs has cost us dearly. We have damaged the ozone layer for decades to come. There has, nevertheless, been a serious attempt to reduce global emissions of CFCs, and other ozone-damaging chemicals, in the shape of the 1987 Montreal Protocol. This has been revised several times in the 1990s and has gone some way toward reducing the problem. However there is still a long way to go, and significant progress towards ozone recovery requires that emissions must be reduced faster than is apparent from current observations in the atmosphere. In the developed world, a large reservoir of CFCs in old refrigeration and vehicle air-conditioning systems continues to leak out, although new CFC production fell nearly fivefold from 1986 to 1995 in accord with the Protocol. Conversely, production is up nearly threefold in the developing world. Nonetheless, technology now exists to recycle or destroy refrigerants that would otherwise leak into the atmosphere when refrigerators are scrapped. Indeed, some chemists are turning their skills to the creation of useful products from unwanted stocks of ozone-depleting chemicals. Although it is not impossible to envisage a route to ozone recovery in the next decades, it will involve much earnest diplomatic effort among the participants of the Montreal Protocol to elicit the necessary level of global stewardship. What must be remembered is that CFCs released even before the Montreal Protocol will still be at work for some time, probably destroying ozone until at least 2090.

With the relative success of the Protocol, it is believed that that the ozone layer will now thin only gradually for ten to twenty years, before it slowly begins to regain its former dimensions. However, at the present time it seems that the ozone hole over the Antarctic is not behaving quite as anticipated. In 2001, the British Antarctic Survey reported that the hole covered 24 million square kilometres, which is more than twice the size of Europe. In size it equals the hole that opened up in 1999, and only the holes in 1998 and 2000 have been larger. In some eyes, because the hole has not grown any larger since 2001, destruction of ozone may have reached a peak. The observations are certainly consistent with the possibility that man-made ozone-destroying chemicals have reached their maximum concentrations in the atmosphere, following the tougher laws regulating their emission and ban on their use in many countries worldwide.

Some chemicals are now getting into the market place labelled as ozone friendly. One of these is *n-propyl bromide*, a new solvent used as a substitute for CFCs. Although a potential ozone destroyer, its survival in the atmosphere was believed to be short, with there being no chance of it reaching the stratosphere. It turns out, however, that if released in the tropics it can reach the stratosphere in a matter of days. Furthermore, it seems that its potential for depleting ozone may be as much as thirty times more in the tropics than in the northern hemisphere. There are still genuine fears that there could yet be many other chemicals in use that could also accumulate in the atmosphere and delay the recovery of the ozone layer. Some candidates have been identified and may be the subject of future legislative restrictions.

## Sunlight and skin

As mentioned in Chapter 1, another type of 'experiment' began in the 1780s. To relieve the problem of overcrowded jails, the British government of the day decided to transport petty criminals to a location as far away as possible. The choice was the east coast of Australia. This area was soon populated with British and Irish descendants, who often shared features of their Celtic origins such as light hair and fair skin. Today they are still the predominant population. These transportations essentially set the scene for a gigantic 'experiment' that established connections between radiation from the sun and its effects on skin.

As many holidaymakers have found out, a day spent too long in the sun can be a painful experience. Warm water becomes scalding hot and towels take on the characteristics of steel wool. When the temperature drops in the evening, even a light jersey does not feel comfortable. 'Sunburn', however, is not burning in the sense of incineration, or heating the skin to abnormal levels. Rather, as you lie comfortably in the warmth of the sun, your skin is not only exposed to visible light but also to two types of ultraviolet radiation: UVA and UVB. It is the UVB that causes the symptoms of sunburn, doing so by triggering the generation of highly reactive free radicals from within the skin. These have to be mopped up before their damaging effects on skin structures get out of control. Fortunately, at the first signs of damage the immune system mounts a rescue operation, sending out various inflammatory chemicals to capture the free radicals, among other things. It is this rapid response that makes skin go red and painful, but only where it has been exposed, hence the clear marks where swimsuits end.

The white population of Australia, with their fair skin continually exposed to powerful sunlight, have more problems than just sunburn. They have the highest incidence of skin cancer of any people in the world. By comparison, their relatives still living in Britain under normally cloudy skies are more fortunate, having a much lower risk of skin cancers. The same is true for Australian Aborigines, who, with their much darker skins, are seldom afflicted by sun-induced cancers of the skin. In fact, the colour of our skin is a major factor in how much we suffer from solar radiation. Darker skins are richer in melanin, a dark brown pigment which acts as a natural sun block. Although the Australian 'experiment' amply demonstrated exposure to strong sun and fair skin to be major risk factors for skin cancer, the actual means whereby sunlight causes skin cells to become malignant took some while to establish.

There are three forms of skin cancer that correspond to the type of skin cell from which they originate. Malignant melanomas arise from melanocytes, cells that normally produce the protective pigment melanin. Although they are the most lethal type of skin cancer, they are fortunately the least common. The two types of non-melanoma skin cancers that arise from the basal and squamous skin cells are more common, but kill only a small proportion of those afflicted.

There is little question that sunlight can kill. Even in the UK, the incidence of malignant melanoma has doubled in the last twenty years and is still escalating. This may be associated with the increasing numbers of people taking holidays in places where the risks are greater than in the UK, where well over 40,000 new cases of skin cancer are now reported each year. The non-melanoma forms account for around 80 per cent of these cancers. Fortunately, those afflicted with these forms of skin cancer have a 97 per cent survival rate, being mainly treatable with surgery under local anaesthesia using freezing or direct excision techniques. It is now clear that solar radiation can penetrate below the surface of the skin to damage sections of our genes that are particularly vulnerable to the ultraviolet light within the sun's rays, the main culprit being UVB radiation (see Table 8.1).

The remaining 20 per cent of skin cancers in the UK are the more dangerous melanomas. These now account for one in twelve cancers in people 15 to 34. In the early stages of development, melanomas can be treated by simple excision, but, unfortunately, later stages require radiotherapy or chemotherapy. The origins of these melanomas reflect sunbathing patterns. In the case of men, the melanomas most often develop on the back or trunk, whereas in women they frequently occur on the leg. Symptoms of melanoma include moles that have changed shape or colour, or have become enlarged, or inflamed with bleeding, ulceration or crusting. The chances of developing melanomas are increased if you have a large number of moles, fair or red hair, a tendency to freckle, a record of severe sunburn episodes (as distinct from tanning), or a history of melanomas in the family. The best cure is prevention. Staying out of the midday sun, wearing a shirt, or T-shirt, and a suitably wide-brimmed hat are recommended. Application of a suitably strong sun block (at least factor 15) will give some short-term protection both from the damaging UVB rays and UVA rays. Another guideline is that when your shadow is shorter than your height, the intensity of the ultraviolet radiation from the sun is most likely to be dangerous.

Although deaths from skin cancers still lag behind those from lung cancer, there is concern that the incidence of skin cancers continues to rise. In the USA, about a million new cases now arise each year. This undoubtedly reflects modern sunbathing habits, and the possibility exists that these statistics may soon be exacerbated by the progressive depletion of the ozone layer.

Although UVB radiation has its serious downside, moderate amounts are nonetheless necessary for the human body to manufacture vitamin D. UVB radiation falling on skin converts a natural chemical in these cells to a form that is transported to the liver and thence to the kidneys. In these organs, it is successively processed into vitamin D. This vitamin is essential for the proper use of calcium in the construction of bone.

## DNA damage and skin cancer

Although skin cancers plague members of all age groups, the critical damage begins many years before the appearance of the cancer, when exposure to the sun's rays caused the modification of a key gene in a single skin cell. Those who emigrated from cloud-covered UK to sun-kissed Australia before the age of 18 appear to suffer skin cancers at a rate similar to the higher incidence of those born in Australia. In contrast, if they emigrated when they were older, their incidence of skin cancer is quite similar to that in the UK. Thus, a critically severe dose of sunlight must have been received some considerable number of years before the appearance of the skin cancers.

Solar radiation can penetrate below the surface of the skin to modify specific nucleotide units of the DNA within skin cells. In particular, DNA is vulnerable to the ultraviolet light within the sun's rays, the main culprit being the UVB rays (see Table 8.1). These rays have the ability first to break chemical bonds within nucleotides that lie next to one another in the strands of DNA, and then create new chemical bonds that bridge these adjacent nucleotides. Most often this occurs between two Ts, (or two Cs, or a T and a C), as illustrated in Figure 8.1.

Such modifications to the nucleotide sequences of skin cells are potentially serious, as the faults, or mutations, can be passed on to progeny cells when the afflicted skin cell divides. Detailed research has now revealed that the majority of squamous cell skin cancers carry a mutation in a particular gene that encodes the information for making a particular protein: *p53*. The same is true in the case of basal cell skin cancers. The protein p53 is important because it has a crucial role in controlling not only the rate at which skin cells normally divide but also how they respond to any damage suffered by their DNA. Normally it functions as a sort of biological brake on the process of cell division. This allows the cell time to carry out running repairs to any

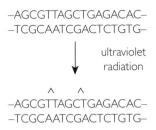

**Figure 8.1**   The way in which ultraviolet radiation can cause adjacent nucleotide units in DNA to become linked together (∧).

damaged DNA before any further cells are propagated (see Chapter 9). However, as will also be explained later (Chapter 10), it can be the case that in skin cells the amount of UVB damage to DNA accumulates to massive proportions. In these situations the p53 protein plays an alternative role, causing that cell to commit suicide. This ensures that no further progeny cells carrying disastrously high numbers of DNA modifications can be propagated and lead to cancers. All of this makes very good sense, but what if the gene that makes p53 is itself modified as a result of attack by UVB radiation? Not surprisingly, this can be serious. The p53 protein made from the altered gene is likely to be defective and may no longer be able to discharge either its repair or its suicide role satisfactorily. Skin cancer cells harbouring such defective p53 proteins are unable to commit suicide and are free to divide in an unregulated style, irrespective of the state of damage to their DNA. While deregulated growth is one of the distinguishing features of cancer cells in general, it still remains to be seen what other genes are involved in the development of skin cancers, particularly malignant melanomas.

## Indirect consequences of ozone loss

The loss of stratospheric ozone could affect our health indirectly. Many animals and plants are also susceptible to the damaging effects of UV rays, thus any rise in UV radiation could harm and upset delicate food chains, which could have serious consequences for human nutrition and welfare in certain parts of the world. Already, research has shown that the productivity of crops such as soya beans and peas deceases by as much as 25 per cent if the UVB content of incident light is increased by a quarter. Recent reports suggest that increased ultraviolet radiation could also be involved in reducing stocks of certain fish by killing their larvae. For instance, Atlantic cod spawn in deep water, but the developing embryos float up towards the surface water to complete their development and could be exposed to potentially damaging levels of radiation.

Although it is possible that the ozone losses will be reversed, we and other organisms clearly face uncertain times.

---

**Key points in this chapter**

- The ozone layer in the stratosphere serves to filter out the most harmful types of solar radiation, and so acts as a first line of defence from its most serious effects.
- Since the 1960s, the ozone layer has been dwindling. A likely culprit is the emission of chlorofluorocarbons (CFCs) into the atmosphere. These are broken down by sunlight, or in reaction with oxygen, to yield chlorine that can destroy ozone.
- As a result of the Montreal Protocol, CFC emissions worldwide are on the wane, and at the present time the dimensions of the ozone hole seem to be remaining fairly constant.
- Excessive sunlight is a serious human health problem at ground level, due to the ability of UVB to initiate various types of skin cancer. Moderate doses of UVB are nonetheless necessary for the formation of vitamin D, required for healthy bone formation.
- Ultraviolet radiation can modify nucleotide units in DNA. It does so by breaking chemical bonds within adjacent nucleotide units and then creating chemical bonds to form a bridge between these neighbouring nucleotides.
- Ultraviolet damage, if it occurs in the gene that makes the protein p53, is central to the initiation of some skin cancers in humans.

# 9

# The main defence forces

The ozone layer does a fairly good job, or at least it did. Up until recently, only around 1 per cent of the sun's potentially dangerous UVB radiation penetrated to the earth's surface; the remainder was screened out. Any increase has to be a matter of concern, and begs the question of whether humans have any inbuilt methods of providing protection from environmental threats. Fortunately, each of us has quite an array of systems that can further act in our defence. Things are better than you might expect from the previous chapters.

From the preceding chapters, it is clear that many types of environmental factor are hazardous to genes because they can bring about chemical alterations to DNA. It is important to realize that such environmentally caused damage is actually superimposed upon an already impressive amount of DNA damage that occurs continuously within cells as a result of natural internal attack, for example from free radicals (see Chapter 7). On this basis, you could not be blamed for being somewhat concerned about the suitability of DNA for its vital role as carrier of genetic information. Without good protection for genes, the continued existence of organisms on this planet would seem under constant threat. However, the fact that life has persisted for so long suggests that there must be other forces at work. In the face of these dangers, in common with other living things, we have evolved quite an impressive array of systems to neutralize, or remove, potentially damaging agents before they have any chance to damage DNA. Important lines of defence include cellular systems for the removal or detoxification of environmental chemicals, as well as mechanisms to scavenge and neutralize free radicals. In addition, we have a further line of defence in the shape of powerful DNA repair systems. By various mechanisms, these can restore the normal nucleotide sequence and structure of DNA, should the initial defence forces be overwhelmed and DNA actually suffer damage.

## Molecular vacuum cleaners

Some cells have a very direct way of neutralizing certain types of potentially toxic chemicals. For example, the membranes that form the boundaries of liver cells contain a special group of *'transporter-type' proteins*. These are capable of collecting and expelling quite a range of diverse chemicals before they can cause any cell damage. The chemicals they can eject even include a number of anticancer drugs. Not surprisingly, this property has the potential to cause considerable problems for clinicians as they attempt to administer life-saving chemotherapy to cancer patients. Rather than taking up some anticancer drugs, the cells targeted in chemotherapy can often become very efficient at expelling them, using such transporters. The transporters are themselves the products of genes which were originally revealed as the explanation for the phenomenon of *multidrug resistance*. In this situation, the patients became resistant not just to one anticancer drug, but to elaborate cocktails. In short, the transporters function as molecular vacuum cleaners, removing certain potentially toxic chemicals, or drugs, from the cell membrane before they can accumulate within cells and do serious damage to cell components such as DNA.

## Many environmental chemicals can be detoxified

We have evolved the ability to neutralize a fair number of potentially toxic environmental chemicals and drugs. An initial objective of the processes, which mainly take place in the liver, is to modify the chemical to a form with increased solubility in water. This is an important prelude to further transformations that enable the offending chemical to be excreted harmlessly in urine. One very important group of liver enzymes that play a crucial role is the cytochrome P450s. Primarily, they can promote the crucial initial transformation of chemicals to more water-soluble forms that we can more readily excrete. When cytochrome P450s were examined in detail, the most striking feature was their diversity. Every individual has a wide variety of different cytochrome P450s and, moreover, the profile of these proteins varies from person to person. This diversity seems to have evolved in response to a variety of environmental challenges that we have experienced in our long evolutionary history. Current estimates range between 60 and 200 different types of cytochrome P450s, classified into ten main groupings. Three of the groups are responsible for neutralizing the potentially harmful effects of a range of environmental chemicals that includes drugs, organic solvents, anaesthetics, dyes, pesticides, alcohols, odorants and flavours. While cytochrome P450s have a clear role in the defence of cells from the ravages of such toxic agents, they nevertheless have a somewhat Jekyll and Hyde character. Depending on the precise structure of the chemical in question, its transformation by cytochrome P450 can instead lead to a product that is highly reactive. Although this can be viewed as an accident of chemistry, it can nonetheless pose serious problems, because, as already mentioned in Chapter 5, such reactive forms can modify certain DNA nucleotide units. Sometimes, in the course of doing their normal job, cytochrome P450s change certain types of chemical, because of their particular structure, into extremely dangerous forms, capable of damaging DNA (see Chapter 5). As already mentioned, there is significant variation between individuals in the range of cytochrome P450s they possess. For example, one type of cytochrome P450 is seen in between 5 and 10 per cent of the Caucasian population, but only in 1 per cent of the Chinese population. Overall, such variation means that individuals will show clear differences, compared with others, in their ability to deal with environmental chemicals, in their conversion either to harmless water-soluble forms, or to highly reactive variants. In short, the susceptibility of humans and their DNA to the range of chemicals in the environment demonstrates considerable genetic diversity.

Cytochrome P450s are not the only means we have at our disposal for decreasing the hazards from potentially toxic chemicals. Another group of cell proteins works by tagging on certain sugar-type molecules to the offending chemical to make it more water-soluble and hence more readily excretable. This type of process is generally known as *conjugation*. Yet another group of proteins achieves detoxification by attaching a molecule called *glutathione* to the toxic chemical. Glutathione itself is a fairly complex molecule found abundantly in all cells. Its normal function is to maintain proteins in the correct chemical state that will allow them to carry out their cell functions. As we shall see shortly, glutathione also has a key role in the defence of cells from the ravages of free radical attack

## Defence against aldehydes

Aldehydes are a common environmental hazard. As will be recalled from Chapter 5, one of this group, formaldehyde, can attack and damage DNA. Formaldehyde in the air is generated from atmospheric methane that originates from decaying plant materials. Other sources include the resins and insulation materials used in the building industry. Formaldehyde and other aldehydes are also products of combustion and are found in cigarette smoke and smog. Foods, especially fruits and vegetables, are notable sources of dietary aldehydes that contribute to flavours and odours. *Malondialdehyde* is present in many foodstuffs; it increases on spoilage and also in microwave-cooked red meats. Aldehydes are also produced in the breakdown of alcohol. Fortunately, we have evolved a variety of proteins capable of converting aldehydes to less reactive forms. Like the cytochrome P450s, they vary considerably within human populations. For example, up to half the Chinese and Japanese populations lack a particular aldehyde-converting protein; alcohol consumption leads to an unwelcome accumulation of acetaldehyde and the development of a characteristic 'alcohol flush'.

## Keeping free radicals at bay

Along with most other organisms, we have gained a significant advantage as a result of the use of oxygen. Mainly this arises because of energy production from food in the complex chain of reactions that takes place inside mitochondria. However, as pointed out in Chapter 7, this use of oxygen does not come without a cost, since there is also a simultaneous, significant generation of unwelcome free radicals during these energy generating processes. These radicals include superoxide radicals, hydroxyl radicals and the related hydrogen peroxide. Living in an atmosphere containing oxygen carries special dangers. It will also be recalled from previous chapters that free radicals are generated within cells, following exposure to environmental hazards such as nuclear radiation and intense sunlight. This is in addition to the free radicals generated from the immune system as it polices the body in the fight against infection.

In common with other organisms living in our oxygen-containing environment, we have evolved a range of specialized defences to protect ourselves from free radical damage. These divide into two classes. First, there are cell proteins whose action promotes the conversion of free radicals, and related species, to harmless entities. Examples of these are *superoxide dismutases* and *catalases*. Second, plant-derived *antioxidants* in food provide another line of defence.

Superoxide dismutases, or SODs for short, turn out to be extremely important to all organisms living in our oxygen-containing environment, as mutant organisms that lack them are extremely sensitive to the toxic effects of oxygen. Recently, alterations to a human gene that encodes an SOD have been detected in patients suffering from a disease called Lou Gehrig's disease or familial amyotrophic lateral sclerosis (FALS). Well-known victims include the eponymous Lou Gehrig, a US baseball star, as well as the world-famous physicist Stephen Hawking. The altered superoxide dismutase that arises from such genes can sometimes cause damage to the nerves carrying impulses from the brain to the skeletal muscles, often leading to paralysis and death.

SODs are the front line of defence against free radical attack. They constitute a family of proteins that convert superoxide radicals into hydrogen peroxide. In addition to possible environmental sources, as already mentioned, significant amounts of superoxide radicals can arise within mitochondria from the chemical processes involved in the generation of energy from food, as well as being released from the cells of the immune system, as they seek out and destroy invading infectious organisms. While this latter source is purpose-built to be lethal to invading bacteria, unfortunately it can sometimes be hazardous for human cells close to a site of infection, as they can be caught in the crossfire. However, there is one group of SODs, found mainly associated with structures on the outsides of cells, that are ideally placed to intercept any superoxide radicals discharged by immune cells in their fight against infectious organisms. The other SODs are to be found within cells. One group is located within mitochondria (see Figure 2.4) and is ideally placed for the capture of superoxide radicals produced there.

Catalases are present in bacteria, plants and animals to promote the transformation of hydrogen peroxide to harmless products. They are extremely efficient at this vital task. A single catalase protein is able to break down more than 40,000 molecules of hydrogen peroxide every second. As mentioned above, hydrogen peroxide can arise from the action of SODs. It can also enter cells in the vicinity of inflammation sites as it is also released from immune cells, because, unlike superoxide radicals, hydrogen peroxide can readily permeate cell membranes. It can be a major hazard for DNA, as highly dangerous hydroxyl radicals can result from its interaction with certain metal ions, such as those from iron or copper, within cell structures.

Hydroxyl radicals, in general, are bad news for all cell structures. Fortunately, we have evolved further means of disposing of hydrogen peroxide. In addition to the very efficient catalases, there are *glutathione peroxidases*. This family of cell proteins is notable because, besides a requirement for glutathione (already mentioned in this chapter), they need an atom of the metal *selenium* to be incorporated into their structure before they will work. This is why we require very small amounts of selenium in our diet and why animals that are deficient in selenium are more susceptible to the toxic effects of high oxygen concentrations than normal. The recommended daily intake of selenium for humans is extremely small, being around 0.000075 grams per day. In Western countries, there is little to worry about as we will usually take in at least that amount in our normal diet. There is, however, a problem. Too much selenium in the diet can be dangerous. Amounts greater than even 0.0003 to 0.0006 grams per day can produce toxic effects such as lack of stamina, in addition to loss of toenails and fingernails and sometimes hair. Food sources especially rich in selenium include whole-wheat grain, liver, kidney, fish and shellfish.

In contrast, there are parts of the Far East where dietary restrictions result in conditions of severe selenium deficiency. In the People's Republic of China there is a degenerative heart condition called Keshan disease, initially detected in a village in the district of Keshan. The symptoms of this condition can be prevented by the administration of small amounts of selenium. Because of this, it is believed that Keshan disease is due to a lack of active glutathione peroxidases. Selenium deficiency may also be at the root of Kasin–Beck disease, which afflicts the joints of children in North China, North Korea and Eastern Siberia. As was the case with Keshan disease, administration of trace amounts of selenium in the diet has considerable beneficial effects. Although an explanation of these diseases is not yet available, it is possible that a build-up of free radicals, due to a lack of glutathione peroxidases, containing the necessary selenium, may be a contributory factor to the symptoms.

## Antioxidants for further protection

Besides these proteins, cells have other devices for keeping free radicals at bay. These come under the general heading of *antioxidants*. In general, these are small molecules that can give away electrons to free radicals and thus reduce their reactivity towards cell components such as DNA. We have already said (in Chapter 7) that free radicals have unpaired electrons and owe their reactivity to a tendency to acquire another electron to make up a pair. To do this, they effectively 'steal' electrons from important cell molecules such as fats, proteins or DNA and leave these cell components in an abnormally unstable state. Antioxidants help to defend these vulnerable cell molecules by donating spare electrons to the attacking free radicals.

One of the main cellular targets for attack by free radicals is the fat-like molecules that are indispensable parts of the membranes surrounding cells (see Figure 2.4). By propagating chain reactions, the free radicals can cause considerable damage. However, *vitamin E*, an antioxidant within cell membranes, can break these chain reactions by virtue of donating electrons to the free radicals involved in the propagation of the membrane damage. In the process, vitamin E itself becomes a free radical, but one which is extremely unreactive, and therefore harmless. It is essential that there is enough vitamin E in cell membranes. Because we cannot make vitamin E ourselves, we must get supplies from our diet. Fortunately, plants make a lot of vitamin E. From a dietary point of view, good sources are vegetable oils, nuts

**Table 9.1**   Relative abundance of vitamin C and carotenoids

| Source | Vitamin C (mg/100 g) | Carotenoids (mg/100 g) |
| --- | --- | --- |
| Orange | 44–79 | 28 |
| Lemon | 58 | 18 |
| Green pepper | 120 | 265 |
| Red pepper | 140 | 3,840 |
| Spinach | 26 | 3,535 |
| Broccoli | 87 | 575 |
| Spring greens | 180 | 2,630 |
| Carrot | 6 | 4,300–11,000 |
| Tomato | 17 | 640 |

*Source*: Adapted from McCance and Widdowson (1992).

and whole grains. Although vitamin E deficiency disease is common among farm animals and can cause severe reproductive problems, acute vitamin E deficiency is rare in humans, as most diets contain adequate amounts.

Vitamin E is converted to a free radical during the process of neutralizing the attacking free radicals, however recent research suggests that vitamin E can be regenerated and return to the fray. The regeneration appears to require *vitamin C*, which itself is an antioxidant, acting directly to scavenge superoxide and hydroxyl radicals. Plants are good sources of vitamin C as is the case with vitamin E. Particularly rich in vitamin C are blackcurrants, peas, potatoes, Brussels sprouts, broccoli, oranges, lemons and kiwi fruit (see also Table 9.1). Like all other primates and guinea pigs we require vitamin C in our diet because we lack the gene that encodes a protein essential for its manufacture. If the diet lacks vitamin C, not only will the antioxidant potential be impaired but we may also develop *scurvy*. Nowadays this condition is rare in developed countries because the consumption of fresh fruits and vegetables has increased. Moreover, most people would

**Table 9.2**    Sources of some flavonoids

| Flavonoid | Source |
| --- | --- |
| Quercitin | Teas, onions, apples, red wine, grapes, berries, broccoli, cranberries |
| Epicatechin gallate | Teas, red wine |
| Chrysin | Fruit skins |
| Myricetin | Berries, grapes, red wine |
| Kaemferol | Endives, leaks, broccoli, radishes, grapefruit, teas |
| Taxifolin | Citrus fruits |
| Apigenin | Celery, parsley |

*Source*: Adapted from Rice-Evans and Miller (1995).

have enough stored vitamin C to provide protection from scurvy for around three months, even if vitamin C became absent from the diet. However, before its importance was realized, vitamin C deficiency caused considerable problems, especially for sailors on long-distance voyages. Poor supplies of vitamin C disrupt the body's normal ability to produce *collagen*. This is a major component of connective tissues that surround our bodies and generally hold them together.

In addition to vitamin C, cells and tissues often contain variable amounts of other antioxidants able to scavenge free radicals. These include *carotenoids* and *flavonoids*. Again, these come from the fruits and vegetables in the diet (see Tables 9.1 and 9.2). At present nearly 600 naturally occurring carotenoids have been identified in an enormous variety of plant sources, one important example being *beta-carotene*, which is present at high concentrations in carrots, but also in dark leafy vegetables, orange and yellow vegetables and yellow fruits (see Table 9.1). Apples, onions, red wine and tea are good sources of the important flavonoid *quercitin* (see also Table 9.2).

Free radicals and green vegetables are now recognized as very important in the context of health. Most people, sensibly, tell their children to 'eat their greens'. As we shall see later, evidence is accumulating that diets rich in fruits and vegetables are associated with longer life expectancy, and it may be that the antioxidants contained therein are of prime importance for these beneficial effects. Certainly, cumulative evidence shows that lower risks of certain cancers and coronary heart disease are associated with diets rich in antioxidant components. Hopefully, the view that salads were invented by women to upset men will be superseded, together with the views of the late Frank Muir, wit and raconteur, who felt that vegetables lacked a sense of purpose and were the also-rans of the dinner plate.

## Human diseases and the repair of DNA

Some twenty years after the discovery of DNA structure, Francis Crick admitted that he had begun to realize that DNA is so precious that there must exist many repair mechanisms to safeguard its integrity. For many, the idea that genes were unstable was deeply worrying. But, going back to the 1930s and early 1940s, there were clear indications, for instance from the work of Alexander Hollaender and his colleagues, that bacteria exposed to X-rays or ultraviolet radiation were capable of some sort of recovery. The crucial role of DNA repair is highlighted by the number of inherited diseases that we now know to be associated with defects in the systems responsible for reacting to DNA damage, or for correcting such damage. These diseases have provided powerful insights into the mechanisms of DNA repair and associated responses in humans.

Since the beginning of the last century, it has been appreciated that various diseases could be passed from parents to offspring. As will be recalled from Chapter 2, one of the earliest of these to be studied in detail was an obscure condition known as alkaptonuria. Otherwise healthy infants with this disease had one striking feature. Their urine rapidly turned black upon exposure to air. In later years they went on to develop arthritis. The dark substance in their urine turned out to be a compound called homogentisic acid. This, as first suggested by the English physician and biochemist Archibald Garrod, is routinely broken down in the tissues of normal people but not in infants with alkaptonuria. The reason for this is that the afflicted infants have inherited faulty copies of a gene from their parents. Normally, this gene encodes information for the construction of a protein that promotes the breakdown of homogentisic acid. However, in situations where the gene is defective, the protein produced from the decoding of the faulty gene is flawed and is unable to carry out its normal function. The result is an abnormal build-up in the infant tissues of homogentisic acid, which ultimately escapes into the urine. Garrod first referred to this type of situation as an 'inborn error of metabolism' and it was soon clear that there were a variety of other inborn errors of metabolism.

By the 1940s it had been shown that the biochemical processes that take place in tissues are genetically controlled; that is to say, each step is directed by a particular protein and, in turn, each specific protein is decoded from one or a few genes. In general, it could be said that if a disease is inherited it is usually caused by an abnormality in a single protein molecule arising from the inheritance of a defective gene. Proteins are of fundamental importance. As pointed out in Chapter 2, almost everything that we do is dependent on the action of one protein or another; life would be impossible without them. For this reason, damage to genes encoding proteins can have a variety of unfortunate consequences for future generations, should the flawed genes be passed on. Sometimes, careful study of the characteristics of the condition that is inherited can shed a great deal of light on the cellular processes in which the defective protein is involved. A particularly important example is the range of protein-based systems that are available within cells which carry out running repairs to DNA and genes, should they suffer damage.

- One of the first human hereditary diseases associated with the repair of damaged DNA to be studied in detail was *xeroderma pigmentosum*. Sufferers are unable to carry out running repairs to DNA damaged in tissues that have been exposed to excessive levels of ultraviolet radiation. As will be recalled from Chapter 8, ultraviolet radiation will cause the breakage of chemical bonds in the nucleotides that lie next to one another in the strands of DNA molecules. New chemical bonds are then formed creating a bridge between these adjacent nucleotides. Fortunately, there are systems within cells that can recognize the occurrence of any such abnormally bridged nucleotides in DNA and take steps to snip them out and to replace that segment of DNA with a fresh, undamaged piece. Victims of xeroderma pigmentosum unfortunately are unable carry this out, as one of the crucial proteins required to excise the damaged section of DNA is itself faulty. Sufferers exhibit an extreme sensitivity to ultraviolet light of the exposed regions of skin, eyes and tongue. Furthermore, they have a high probability of developing skin cancers as well as neurological disorders.

- Another hereditary disease that is characterized by an inability to repair ultraviolet-damaged DNA is *trichothiodystrophy*. Most of these patients are abnormally sensitive to ultraviolet light, as well as having sulphur-deficient, brittle hair and skin scales. They also show physical and mental retardation.

- Victims of *Cockayne syndrome* are another group that cannot repair ultraviolet-damaged DNA. They are characteristically dwarfed, and are also highly sensitive to ultraviolet light.

- Patients that have inherited *Fanconi's anaemia* cannot repair DNA that has become damaged as a result of interstrand cross-linking (see Chapter 5). Clinically, the disease is complex, but primarily it is characterized by a depression in the level of blood cells, together with diverse congenital abnormalities. Additionally, victims have an increased risk of leukaemia and solid tumour development and their cells have an elevated level of chromosome aberrations.

- Besides cross-linking and ultraviolet damage, another type of DNA damage that cells normally attempt to repair is strand breakage, such as would be encountered, for example, in tissues exposed to ionizing radiation (see Chapter 3). Some clues as to the cell systems involved have come from the study of patients with *ataxia telangiectasia*, or AT for short. These patients have symptoms that include deficiencies in their immune responses, growth retardation, and roughly a hundredfold increase in the incidence of cancers, particularly those originating in cells that act as precursors to mature white blood cells. The cells of AT patients are hypersensitive to ionizing radiation and other agents that induce DNA strand breaks, suggesting that they are unable to recognize, or repair, this type of DNA damage. In particular they are slow to raise levels of the cell protein p53. As will be recalled from the previous chapter, this important cell protein plays a key role in controlling the rate at which cells proliferate and how they respond to damage in their DNA. Usually the protein p53 acts as a sort of biological handbrake on the process of cell division, in order to allow the cell time to carry out running repairs to any damaged DNA before any further cells are propagated. AT patients appear to have inherited a flawed gene, which, in its normal form, encodes a protein that either functions alone in the repair of DNA strand breaks, or in conjunction with the protein p53, in the cell division control mechanisms that operate in response to such DNA damage.

- AT is not the only heritable disease in which victims display an inability to repair DNA strand breaks. Sufferers from *Nijmegen breakage syndrome* have deficiencies in their immune systems and an increased propensity to develop cancers of the blood. Although many of their symptoms overlap with those of AT patients, there are no neurological signs. Features of this condition include a high degree of sensitivity to ionizing radiation and inability to control the cell division processes. The faulty gene that is inherited by these patients normally encodes a protein called *nimbrin* that plays a role in linking the repair of DNA strand breaks (particularly double strand breaks) with the control of cell proliferation.

- Finally, one of the most common human cancer susceptibility conditions is also associated with inherited defects in the ability to repair DNA. This is known as *hereditary non-polyposis colon cancer*. The DNA alteration that is inherited by victims is in a gene whose protein product normally participates in the removal and repair of improperly paired nucleotides. Although colon cancers are the main type of cancer seen in these patients, 35 to 40 per cent develop a range of other cancers.

Overall, the fact that there is a number of well-established heritable human diseases characterized by serious defects in the ability to repair damaged DNA underscores the fundamental importance of DNA repair mechanism to our general good health. A key point to emerge, and one to which we shall return, is that defects in the genes for proteins involved in DNA repair processes appear to increase our chances of developing cancers.

## How is DNA repaired?

Although present knowledge of the mechanisms available to cells to patch up damaged DNA is far from complete, the fact that established human diseases manifest deficiencies in DNA repair has already contributed greatly to our general understanding of the processes involved. Complementary information has come from other studies carried out with various bacteria and other microbes. In general, it is now known that a variety of distinct systems exist within cells to carry out different sorts of DNA repair work. Some details of these are given below.

- One system comprises proteins that are capable of directly reversing certain very simple types of modification that have occurred to DNA nucleotide units. These *alkyltransferases*, however, are very limited in their scope.
- Another type of system, which can involve as many as thirty different proteins, is called *nucleotide excision repair*. It first snips out a segment of the DNA strand containing the damaged nucleotide or nucleotides. The proteins of this system then replace the faulty section with a new piece of DNA. Overall, this system can deal with a wide range of chemical modifications to DNA, as well as the nucleotide damage caused by ultraviolet light and free radicals.
- In yet another type of excision repair system, *base excision repair*, instead of cutting out a sizeable segment of DNA containing the damaged nucleotide, only a small part of the damaged nucleotide itself is excised before the overall structure of the DNA is made good. This system is generally involved in the repair of DNA that has become altered spontaneously or damaged by ionizing radiation and/or free radicals.
- *Mismatch repair systems* are also available to correct nucleotide units that have been erroneously inserted into DNA. This can happen during the copying process, or nucleotide units can become incorrectly matched due to certain types of DNA damage. It is one of the proteins involved in this particular repair system that has been found to be faulty in the human disease hereditary nonpolyposis colon cancer.
- *Double-strand break repair* is also possible. This would be a necessity in the case of severe damage to DNA from ionizing radiation. One

possibility is that a certain amount of such damage can be repaired by very intricate systems in which nucleotide sequence information lost from the damaged DNA on one chromosome of a pair is retrieved by exchange with information from the partner chromosome that remains undamaged (remember, each cell contains pairs of chromosomes).

Despite this impressive array of specialized systems dedicated to the repair of different types of DNA damage, it is important to realize that they are not perfect and can be overwhelmed depending on the severity of the exposure to a particular hazard. As pointed out in Chapter 7, continuous attack on DNA from free radicals generated within cells is already extensive, and external environmental factors produce further damage. The efficiency of the different DNA repair systems is also variable. Sometimes, if a certain type of DNA damage is particularly severe, it might not get repaired due to the relative inefficiency of the particular system involved. Damage remaining unrepaired can be lethal to a cell, as it can make the copying of its DNA impossible. If copying is still possible, some types of DNA damage can lead to mistakes during the copying process, such as the insertion of incorrect nucleotides into the progeny DNA molecules. These are subsequently perpetuated as mutations, or hereditable alterations in the nucleotide sequence of DNA. As we shall see later in this book, some mutations can have considerable consequences in terms of health and disease, and even in the process of ageing.

---

**Key points in this chapter**

- Cells are equipped with a variety of different systems that can reduce the hazards to DNA from a range of environmental chemicals.
- Some systems comprise proteins within cell membranes that can directly expel toxic chemicals from cells before they can accumulate to dangerous levels.
- Other systems act to increase the water solubility of many toxic chemicals, and thus our ability to excrete them in urine.

- We can limit the potential for free radical attack on DNA and genes. Cells have proteins that can alter superoxide radicals and hydrogen peroxide, thus limiting the opportunity within cells for the generation of free radicals.
- Other defences against free radicals include dietary antioxidants. These can readily give electrons away to free radicals, neutralizing their dangerous reactivity.
- We also have an impressive array of systems for repairing damage to DNA and genes caused, for instance, by nuclear and ultraviolet radiations and toxic chemicals.
- Human heritable diseases exist in which the victims are unable to carry out running repairs to their DNA. These diseases are due to faults in genes that encode one or more of the proteins that comprise the repair systems.
- A notable feature of patients with hereditable diseases of DNA repair is their higher than normal chances of developing cancer.

# What if our defences are overwhelmed?

The new techniques of genetic engineering have made it possible to create laboratory mice that lack the genetic information for certain types of DNA repair. These mice turn out to be extremely sensitive to agents that damage DNA. Moreover, they show many signs of premature ageing and they readily develop cancers. Such abnormalities attest to the crucial importance of DNA repair systems in protecting organisms from DNA damage.

## To die or not to die

DNA damage is particularly threatening to cells during the processes of DNA copying and subsequent cell division. The process of copying itself could make the damage irreparable, and ensuing cell division can sometimes lead to gross chromosomal abnormalities in the progeny cells. To combat this menace, our cells employ a mechanism that can temporarily halt cell division, should any DNA damage be detected. This provides a vital breathing space for the necessary repairs to be carried out. Many of the signals in cells that relay information about DNA damage are channelled through a key cellular component already mentioned, namely the protein p53 (see Chapters 8 and 9). This protein is a kind of emergency handbrake on the processes of cell division. Not only can p53 orchestrate the necessary interruption to cell division, it can also signal up the appropriate DNA repair machinery. In general, the ultimate effectiveness of DNA repair varies considerably with the nature of the damage inflicted; some forms are simply more difficult to repair than others.

Despite systems that put the brakes on cell division in the face of repairable DNA damage, it now appears that serious, and possibly irreparable, damage may cause the p53 protein to circumvent the cell division blocking systems and, instead, trigger a process known as *apoptosis* (also referred to as *programmed cell death*). By this means, tissues can be purged of cells whose DNA, if copied, might contain aberrations sufficient to cause cancers. A potentially serious situation for health would develop if, for some reason, the p53 protein were faulty, thus preventing the eradication of such cells.

Apoptosis has, in fact, been recognized for some time as a normal process of cell removal, operating as an essential component of normal tissue housekeeping. As you read this, millions of your cells are committing suicide, but this isn't a cause for undue concern. The bulk of this self-sacrifice is to ensure survival. Your health depends not only on your ability to produce new cells, but also on the ability of individual cells to self-destruct when they become superfluous to requirements, or become deranged in some critical way. The process of cell suicide is integral to the building of tissues during development from infancy, as well as the functioning of tissues during adult life. By the 1950s, researchers who studied the way embryos develop found that animals attained their final form by eliminating selected cell types at various specific stages on the way. For instance, the tadpole deletes its tail during transformation into a frog; and mammals erase countless neurones as their nervous systems take shape. Although most of the observable events that define apoptosis, together with its role in the development of embryos, were first noted in the 1950s, it is only recently that the importance of apoptosis in the daily maintenance of fully formed adult organisms has been appreciated. In a seminal paper of 1972, John Kerr, an Australian pathologist, and his Scottish colleagues Andrew Wyllie and Alistair Currie, argued that the type of programmed cell death that occurs during embryo development also occurs in mature organisms and, importantly, carries on throughout their life. It is a deliberate and genetically programmed response by cells, and its failure can contribute to the onset of cancers. The name 'apoptosis' is derived from classical Greek, meaning 'dropping off', as in the dropping of flower petals or falling leaves. Overall, the process is a subtly orchestrated disassembly of critical cell structures, permitting unwanted cells to vanish with the minimum of disruption to surrounding tissues. It is characterized by the controlled condensation of the cell nucleus and cytoplasm and the fragmentation of DNA. This programmed cell death, or apoptosis, can be distinguished from *necrotic cell death*, which occurs when a cell is severely injured, for example following a physical blow, or by oxygen deprivation. Unlike apoptosis, necrotic cell death is not genetically programmed.

## Mutation

Cells and tissues resemble a fortress under siege. They can repel many threats from external forces, but occasionally the severity of the on-slaught may be such that even the impressive lines of defence, made up of antioxidants, various detoxifying enzymes and DNA repair systems, are inadequate and can be breached. In such situations, damage can be inflicted on genes. External agents are not the only sources of danger. Internally generated free radicals can also breach cell defences and cause significant harm to DNA (see Chapter 7). Estimates of the extent of this particular risk vary, but there has been a suggestion that it could be a high as 10,000 hits on the DNA of each of our cells every day. The cellular DNA repair systems nevertheless make good most of this damage, although, at any one time, it is possible to detect around 150,000 nucleotides unrepaired out of the cellular total of 3 billion. Ultimately, the level of injury to DNA is dependent not only on the severity of the assault but also on the effectiveness of the overall defence capability available within cells and tissues.

As might be anticipated, when the copying machinery tries to deal with damaged DNA, mistakes are made, and progeny cells result with aberrations in their DNA nucleotide sequences. The problem does not stop there, as these errors in turn can be passed faithfully on to future generations of cells. Generally speaking, all types of heritable altera-tions in DNA nucleotide sequences, whatever their cause, are referred to as mutations; *mutagen* is the name given to an agent that increases the frequency of such heritable changes. As we shall see later, although mutations have been essential to evolution, they can have serious consequences in the shorter term in relation to genetic diseases and cancer, as well as in ageing.

There are different types of mutation. Some only involve the replacement of a single nucleotide in a DNA sequence with another. Others amount to the deletion or addition of nucleotides to the normal sequence. In some more extreme cases, quite extensive lengths of a DNA sequence may become repeated, or even relocated elsewhere in a chromosome. In general, these heritable changes in DNA nucleotide sequences can have consequences for decoding processes that turn the DNA nucleotide sequence information into the proteins required for cell functions. As we saw in Chapter 2, a defect in the sequence of DNA that represents a gene could specify an error in the amino acid sequence of the particular protein encoded by that gene. Because of its aberrant amino acid sequence, this 'mutated' protein may no longer be capable of discharging its usual role.

With our developing ability to isolate and determine the precise order of nucleotides within individual genes, it is now possible to examine specific mutations and the factors that cause them. Which genes are the most vulnerable? Which locations within these genes are most prone to mutation, occurring either spontaneously or in response to known environmental factors? The answers to these questions is highly relevant to the problems of human genetic disease, as well as to the development of cancers and the processes of ageing. The frequency of mutation can vary greatly from one gene to another. Spontaneous mutation has been observed to occur in certain types of DNA sequences at very much higher rates than is the case for other regions. These are often referred to as mutational 'hot spots'. Often they are made up of runs of identical nucleotides, or short nucleotide sequences that are extensively repeated. Such unusual sites could readily gain nucleotides by accidental slippage of the copying mechanism during the DNA replication process.

## Mutations and the environment

What influence can the environment have on mutations, the basic mechanism for genetic change? Since the 1930s, it has been appreciated that certain environmental factors can influence mutation rates. For example, at that time it was found that exposure of experimental animals and microorganisms to ionizing radiation can have dramatic effects on the mutation rate. The *Ames* test was an early test for the ability of environmental chemicals to cause mutations, based on their ability to bring about mutations in special strains of Salmonella bacteria. The test was constructed to indicate whether a chemical would cause mutations *directly* in the test bacteria, or *indirectly* after transformation by cytochrome P450 to a reactive form, capable of modifying DNA, as described in Chapters 5 and 9. While many types of bacterial mutagenicity tests have been developed over the years, their greatest use has been in classifying chemicals according to their biological activity, monitoring environmental samples and predicting possible toxicological effects.

Studies on the distribution of mutations within the nucleotide sequences of known genes have revealed specificities that are characteristic of different mutagens. For example, ultraviolet radiation will elicit types of mutation that are different from those produced by the food contaminant aflatoxin B1, and those caused by the PAH benzpyrene and so on. Although different mutagens exhibit specificity with regard to the type of mutation they cause, the rates at which these mutations occur appear to be affected by the nature of the DNA nucleotide sequences in the vicinity. Some sequences are more likely to suffer mutation than others. In part, this could reflect the three-dimensional organization of chromosomal DNA within cell nuclei. Some regions of DNA may simply be more readily accessible to the mutagen than others. Additionally, the overall mutation rate at a specific DNA location may reflect the rate at which the type of damage at that position can be repaired.

A number of recent investigations have focused on mutations associated with key genes. One particular gene that has received a great deal of attention is the one encoding the protein p53. As described previously, this crucial protein functions not only as an emergency brake on cell division in the face of DNA damage, but also as part of the triggering mechanism that initiates programmed cell death (apoptosis), should DNA be beyond repair. Mutations in the gene for p53 can thus have serious consequences for these vital processes. Moreover, as we shall see later, mutations in the p53 gene are also implicated in the development of most human cancers. The length of the complete gene for p53 corresponds to around 20,000 nucleotide units; four separate mutational hot spots can be detected. These correspond to regions that specifically code for the exact parts of p53 crucial for its function in relation to DNA damage. One of the hot spots is regularly found in a mutated form in victims of liver cancer. This condition occurs extensively in China, where the food contaminant aflatoxin B1 is a notable risk factor.

Our extensive knowledge of mutations affecting the gene for p53 has been gathered from the examination of DNA samples taken from tumour samples taken at post-mortems. This has its limitations. At present, it is not possible to monitor continuously the status of the p53 gene in cells of people, like cigarette smokers, who, although still alive, may be at risk of developing lung cancer. On the other hand, it is possible to examine the DNA from regularly taken blood samples for mutations in the p53 gene and other key genes. This could provide evidence of a pattern of mutation that may indicate exposure to particular mutagenic environmental agents and an indication of the extent of likely damage. Samples of blood are removed and from these are isolated a group of blood cells called T-cells. These can be grown in a laboratory to provide a source of DNA sufficient in quantity to do the necessary nucleotide sequence analyses. When this has been done, the frequency of mutations observed in many genes has been shown to increase with the age of the subject, although it is also further elevated in tobacco smokers, and in individuals undergoing radiotherapy and chemotherapy. Despite these complications, recognition of particular patterns of mutation in specific genes from the DNA of possible victims would be a means of identifying the nature of the potential cancer-causing agent involved.

## The problem of cancer

One of the least acceptable features of mutation is cancer. Over the world the incidence of different cancers varies widely. For those living in Scotland there are particular risks. The cancer rates there are now the worst in the UK, being around a fifth higher than those in England. Lung and bowel cancer are more prevalent, both being major killers, accounting for nearly 600 deaths a year in Scotland. There is a high incidence of skin cancer in Australia, of oesophageal cancer in Iran, of stomach cancer in Japan, of liver cancer in Mozambique and Kenya, and rectal cancer in Denmark. There seems to be a strong connection between the environment and cancer. This is supported by cancer incidence rates in populations that emigrate from one environment to another. People who emigrated from Japan to the United States as children have incidences of various cancers that more closely reflect those in the United States than those in Japan. In Japan, stomach cancer is much more common than in the United States, but cancers of the of the large intestine, breast and prostate are less common.

According to recent statistics, four out of ten people living in the UK will develop cancer in their lifetime. On the face of it, things seem to be getting worse – only fifteen years ago, three people in ten were at risk of developing the disease in the UK. One explanation put forward is that we are living to an older age, when the disease is more common. However, there are other factors that should not be discounted. Almost 1,000 to 1,500 new chemicals are being introduced into the environment each year, of which no more than a minor fraction are tested for cancer connections.

Although cancer is a scourge primarily of the Western world, the Third world is catching up: cases there are likely to double by 2020. Despite the fact that billions of pounds have been spent in searches for cures, the overall death rate from cancers still rises. On a brighter note, although more of us are getting cancer, our chances of surviving longer have never been better, early detection being a significant factor.

While most types of cancer show little tendency to run in families, it is now clear that the disease can have a genetic element. Cancers are not passed on directly from generation to generation through sperm and eggs. Their origins appear to involve mutations in other cell types, such as those in lungs, liver, kidney, pancreas and skin, the so-called *somatic cells*. Many different types of environmental factors including solar radiation, nuclear radiation, air pollutants, tobacco smoke and chemicals can cause these *somatic mutations*. Some somatic mutations have life-threatening consequences, causing the orderly succession of somatic cell divisions to go awry, so contributing to the development of cancers.

The increased frequency of mutations in the somatic cells of the victims is a significant characteristic of a number of hereditary diseases associated with defective repair of DNA damage (see Chapter 9). This is accompanied by a heightened susceptibility to the development of cancers. Even if we are not afflicted with these diseases, we nonetheless accumulate an increasing number of somatic mutations as we grow older. Although many of these accumulated mutations are likely to be the result of a lifetime's exposure to assorted external environmental factors, they could also accrue as a consequence of attack from sources within cells themselves. Whatever their origin, such accumulated mutations will also increase our chances of developing cancers.

## How does cancer develop?

A normal healthy human cell responds to the dictates of the environment within its tissue. It only gives rise to progeny cells when the balance of stimulatory and inhibitory growth signals that come to it from various sources in the body indicate that division should take place. It is this process, with its requirement to copy the cell's DNA, that carries the hazard of passing on any unrepaired defects such as mutations. Some of these could undermine the delicate regulatory networks that control the processes of cell division. A single mutation may be sufficient to allow a cell to undergo the occasional unscheduled division and be less responsive to the dictates of the normal growth signals coming to it. If such mutations accumulate, progeny cells that are totally unresponsive to such external growth control signals may ultimately be generated. No longer will such cells respond to growth inhibitory signals; instead they gain the ability to divide uncontrollably and may exhibit signs of malignancy. In this state the resulting mass of cells not only can impinge on, and damage, adjacent healthy tissues but can also cross the barriers between one organ and another, and thereby *metastasize*. That is, they can set up colonies at sites within the victim's body, which may be quite distant and different from their origin. For example, cancer cells originating in the lung can enter the bloodstream and metastasize to other sites such as liver, brain and bones, and, once there, proceed to divide further, producing an even greater tumour mass.

If the level of mutations in somatic cells increases as we grow older, it is reasonable to ask whether there are any types of mutations that are particularly relevant to cancer development, because not everyone gets cancers as they age. One group of mutations that are central to the development of cancers are those occurring within a class of genes called the *protooncogenes*. These code for proteins that normally facilitate cell division. Some sit on the surfaces of cells and have the specific job of receiving incoming growth signal molecules sent to the cell from other tissues of the body. When these signals are received, the cell surface proteins send signals to the interior of the cell. Other cell proteins, also coded for by protooncogenes, are involved in further relaying the growth signal to systems within cells that are responsible for the initiation of cell division. When mutations occur in proto-oncogenes, they become known as *oncogenes*. Crucially, the proteins produced from these altered genes no longer tightly control the process of cell division. A mutated protooncogene might overproduce a growth regulatory protein, or produce a faulty version that is inappropriately active. It might transmit false signals within cells, even when no normal growth signals had been sent. Indeed, the hyperactive products of a certain mutated protooncogene, called *ras*, can be found in 25 per cent of all human cancers, including those of the colon, pancreas and lung. Although the conversion by mutation of individual protooncogenes to oncogenes can initiate the deregulation of cell division, by themselves they are unable to cause cancers. Another group of genes called tumour suppressor genes is usually required, as will be explained later.

## Predisposition to cancer

Although most forms of cancer do not run in families, there are nonetheless two classes of mutation which can be inherited and pre-dispose that person to the possibility of developing cancers. We have already encountered one group of these: the mutations afflicting the genes that encode DNA repair systems, as in the heritable diseases xeroderma pigmentosum, Fanconi's anaemia, and ataxia telangiectasia. If DNA repair is faulty, then the number of mutations passed on to progeny cells during the process of tumour development may increase substantially. In turn, the progeny cells may then pass on DNA carry-ing even more mutations to their progeny. Defects in genes for DNA repair proteins may simply increase the speed at which certain tumours arise and become life-threatening. Another condition belonging to this group of DNA repair deficiency diseases is hereditary non-polyposis colon cancer, one of the most common human cancer-susceptibility conditions known. Although colon cancers are the main types of cancer that develop in these patients, a number of these victims go on to develop other types of cancer.

A second class of mutations conferring susceptibility to cancer development occur in genes that direct the manufacture of proteins whose function is the suppression of cell division. These are also known as the *tumour suppressor genes*. Mutations that result in the loss of the suppressor characteristics of their protein products can set cells free of restraints on the frequency of their division. A well-known example of a tumour suppressor gene is that encoding the protein p53, already mentioned a number of times. Mutations leading to the absence of functional p53 are found in half of all types of human cancers.

Further evidence for the existence of tumour suppressor genes came from studies of rare types of cancers that run in families. Members of affected families appear to inherit susceptibility to cancer and develop certain particular kinds of tumours at rates much higher than the normal population. A dramatic example of inherited tumour suscepti-bility is *retinoblastoma*, a tumour of the eye that strikes young children. Around a third of retinoblastoma patients develop multiple tumours, usually in both eyes. Furthermore, the children and siblings of such patients often develop the same disease. At the root of this condition are mutations in a suppressor gene that encodes the so-called *retino-blastoma protein*. This protein turns out to have a much wider signifi-cance, and, like p53, in its non-mutated form is involved in the cellular mechanisms that suppress cell division. If mutated, this suppressor function is lost. Although mutations in the gene for retinoblastoma protein gene were originally detected in patients who developed retino-blastoma, recent studies have also found such mutations in patients who develop cancers of the lung, bladder, bone and breast.

Studies on the development of breast cancer have also indicated the possible involvement of genes that confer increased susceptibility. Although one women in twelve in the UK develops breast cancer, such tumours appear mostly to be driven by the female sex hormone oestrogen, with the disease usually striking around the age of 50 or over. It is not so common in young women, unless they carry mutated forms of genes called *BRCA-1* and *BRCA-2*. The precise role of these breast cancer susceptibility genes is still the subject of much investigation, but the normal form of BRCA-1 seems to act as a tumour suppressor gene, and its protein product may be involved in the control of cell division. Women with a mutation in BRCA-1 inherit a 60 per cent probability of developing breast cancer before the age of 50. In non-inherited breast cancer, BRCA-1 is generally not mutated.

## Cancer progression

It is now clear that cancer development involves the progressive accumulation, in one cell and its direct descendants, of mutations in both tumour suppressor genes and protooncogenes. In the first instance, a single cell might suffer a mutation in a protooncogene or a tumour suppressor gene that allows it to divide under conditions which normally prevent cells from dividing. The next generation of cells derived from these inappropriately dividing cells carries the same mutation, and exhibits the same aberrant growth characteristic. Some time later, one of these cells or their descendants suffers another mutation, either in a protooncogene or tumour suppressor gene, that further enhances its ability to evade normal regulation. This additional mutation is passed to progeny cells. Repetition of this general sequence of events, referred to as *clonal expansion*, allows one original cell, and its direct progeny, to accumulate a variety of specific mutations. In addition to those mutations in protooncogenes or tumour suppressor genes, other genes can also be mutated so that the cells can pass through normal tissue barriers, enter the bloodstream and metastasize in other organs of the body.

To put these events in a particular context, consider the development of cancers of the colon, which has been particularly well studied. One of the earliest detectable mutations occurs in a suppressor gene called *APC*. This appears to cause a relaxation in the normal rigorous control of DNA copying. Colon cancers also carry mutations in two other suppressor genes, one of which encodes the p53 protein. On top of these, a mutation in the protooncogene called *ras* is also detectable in the DNA from colon tumours. Although the mutation in ras occurs early in the progression to malignancy, the precise order in which the mutations relevant to the development of colon cancers occur has not yet been established.

In many laboratories around the world, the mutations in suppressor genes and protooncogenes relating to the development of different types of cancer are now being intensively studied. As already mentioned, mutations in suppressor genes encoding p53 and retinoblastoma protein occur in a considerable proportion of cancer types. In addition, the mutations that were originally detected in hereditary non-polyposis colon cancer now appear to occur in about 0.5 per cent of the human population as a whole and can dramatically increase the risk not only of colon cancer but also of ovarian, uterine and kidney cancers.

Clinically, many different types of cancer are recognized. They are classified according to the tissue and cell type from which they arise. There are some broad categories. For instance those that arise from epithelial cells (the cells that line the surfaces of organs and body cavities) are referred to as *carcinomas*, whereas those arising from connective tissue or muscle cells are called *sarcomas*. Others, such as *leukaemias*, are derived from cells that are precursors to blood cells. If the dividing cancer cells remain at their site of origin as a discrete mass, they are said to be *benign* and can usually be removed from the patient by surgery. The term *malignant* refers to tumours that have reached a state of development where they break loose from their original sight of development and metastasize at other sites in the body.

## Cancers develop over a long timescale

From the initial mutation in a single cell to the development of a full-blown malignant cancer may take as long as fifteen to twenty years. This is extremely important when considering any possible link between environmental factors and cancer development. Lung cancer does not usually manifest itself until after some ten to twenty years of heavy smoking, and the occurrence of leukaemias did not increase in Japan until around five to eight years after the atomic blasts of 1945.

Furthermore, workers in industries where they were exposed for limited periods to carcinogenic chemicals did not develop cancers until some ten to twenty years after the initial exposure. As already emphasized, a single mutation, even in a protooncogene or suppressor gene, is insufficient to cause cancer. Cancers develop in slow stages and it has been estimated that, for humans, around five to seven independent mutations in protooncogenes and suppressor genes are necessary for the development of a malignant cancer. A good proportion of these may inevitably accumulate in the relevant genes within somatic cells, either as a result of exposure to environmental mutagens or as a simple function of ageing. Alternatively, some persons may inherit mutations from parents. With a number of mutations already on board, such people can manifest a greater susceptibility to cancers than the rest of the population. This may simply be because the number of additional mutations that have to be accumulated in the somatic cells of these persons is much lower than would be the case normally.

## Does mutation contribute to ageing?

Although environmental factors can be significant in the development of cancers because they can cause mutations in protooncogenes and suppressor genes, their general ability to cause mutations in somatic cells may also be very relevant to the overall processes of ageing. All of us are exposed, throughout our lives, to DNA-damaging agents, not only from environmental sources but also from internal sources, such as the free radicals from immune cells and mitochondria. Indeed, some gerontologists now believe that this constant exposure to such oxygen-related free radicals may be central to the transformations associated with ageing. Although various antioxidant defences have evolved to combat this persistent threat, these are not perfect, and as we age our DNA accumulates free radical damage. On top of this, our ability to repair DNA damage decreases with age. This is particularly evident in individuals with *Werner's syndrome*, a rare heritable disease with some of the symptoms of premature ageing. The defective gene in these patients is one which, in its normal form, encodes a protein that is probably connected with DNA repair processes. For these reasons, it is perhaps not surprising that mutations accumulate in our DNA as we age, as does the rate of mutation. One example of this is that the rate of mutation in the DNA of white blood cells (lymphocytes) is some ninefold higher in adults than in newborn infants.

It has been argued that general free radical damage to cell structures is a cause of ageing. Exposure of experimental animals to ionizing radiation, which generates free radicals from the water within tissues, can reduce their lifespan and cause changes similar to those encountered in normal ageing. In addition, it has been observed that animals with higher tissue levels of antioxidants, such as vitamin E and carotenoids, have greater life expectancy. Another approach has been to reduce the calorie content of animals' diets. This also increases their lifespan. As will be recalled, the mitochondria within cells are responsible for the conversion of food into energy. However, the processes involved can also generate superoxide radicals. These may well contribute significantly to the ageing of the animals, and a reduced food intake would be expected to diminish such free radical production. The *free radical hypothesis of ageing* has been advanced as a means of explaining the cumulative changes resulting in the increased possibility of death as age increases. It could simply be the price we have to pay for living in an atmosphere containing oxygen and using free radicals in our immune systems as protection from invasion by infectious organisms.

There are more specific views on the mechanisms of ageing. For instance, another view is that, because mitochondria are primary sites within our cells for the generation of free radicals, damage to the components of mitochondria themselves is a critical factor in ageing. Such damage could impair the efficiency of the mitochondrial energy-generating systems and give rise to even greater superoxide radical production, leading to eventual cell and tissue malfunction that could contribute to the symptoms of ageing.

A quite different view is that we may have *longevity genes*. Some research has shown that mutant worms, which are especially long-lived, appear to have mutations in genes whose products are involved in determining their normal lifespan. However, one particular mutant of this type had elevated levels of the antioxidant defence enzymes superoxide dismutase and catalase, and accumulated DNA damage at a reduced level compared with normal worms. It appears that the free radical theory of ageing and concepts based on longevity genes may well have some common features. The mutant worms were also more resistant to a range of environmental stresses, including ultraviolet radiation and elevated temperatures. The lifespan of fruit flies has also been deliberately extended by use of genetic engineering techniques to increase their levels of superoxide dismutase and catalase. These and other studies suggest that lifespan is under some sort of regulatory control that results from the alteration of the sensitivity of the organism to the environment, together with an increased ability to resist or repair environmental damage. Stress tolerance may well be the key to a longer life.

---

**Key points in this chapter**

- Excessive DNA damage can lead to programmed cell death (apoptosis), thus protecting us from cells whose DNA is severely damaged.
- Less extensive DNA damage (or modification) that escapes repair can be perpetuated during the copying processes as mutations in future cell generations.
- Mutagens are agents which increase the rate at which mutations occur.
- Analysis of the location of mutational 'hot spots' may be a way to establish relationships between different environmental agents and specific genetic changes.
- There is a strong connection between the environment and cancer.
- Although most forms of cancer do not run in families, it is possible to inherit increased susceptibility to certain cancers. Victims of heritable diseases that manifest deficiencies in DNA repair are also more susceptible to the development of cancer.
- Mutations in protooncogenes and tumour suppressor genes are linked to the development of cancers.
- The timescale of cancer development can be as long as twenty years.
- The progressive accumulation of unrepaired gene damage may contribute to the process of ageing.

# Can we survive the siege?

Cancer is a very serious consideration. Around 30,000 women in the UK die of breast cancer every year. As a whole, the disease is now striking the general population at a rate that is increasing at 1 per cent per annum. Today, cancer kills one man in two and one woman in three. However, it is estimated that at least 80 per cent of cancers are likely to be due to environmental factors that could be either eradicated or reduced. Industrialized countries seem to have disproportionately more cancers than countries with few industries, and studies on populations that migrate from underdeveloped to developed countries indicate that it is the new environment that determines the risk rather than the genetic background. Particularly notable are the increases in breast and lung cancer, multiple myeloma, melanoma and non-Hodgkin's lymphoma, although cancers of the prostate, testes, kidney and larynx have also risen. While cancer is mainly thought of as a disease of old age, childhood leukaemias have also shown a disturbing increase (some 20 per cent between 1950 and 1988).

## Cancer epidemiology

Over the last fifty years or so, epidemiologists have sought to evaluate environmental causes of cancer. Their task is to identify factors that are common to cancer victims' histories and ways of life and evaluate them in the context of our current biological and medical knowledge. They attempt to decide whether exposure to certain factors, or personal behaviour characteristics, significantly increases the odds of particular cancers developing. Work of this type has thrown light on many of the environmental causes of cancer and also provided estimates of the annual number of deaths attributable to each. There is a wealth of research to link cancers with what we eat, drink and breathe. Cancer has been compared to the Black Death as the plague of the twentieth century. Its emergence parallels the gradual industrialization of the world, and the widespread introduction of new synthetic chemicals into the workplace.

A great deal of knowledge has been accumulated, unfortunately often at great cost in terms of human life, regarding the cancer-causing potential of a large number of dangerous substances encountered in the environment, particularly the workplace. Well-known examples include tobacco smoke, asbestos, formaldehyde, diesel exhaust, benzene and radon. This information now forms the basis of the legislative control of many occupational hazards in the workplace. In the developed world at least, increasingly rigorous control measures over the last fifty years have halved the proportion of cancer deaths caused by occupational exposure. Recent estimates suggest that around 40 carcinogens now contaminate drinking water, while 60 or so are released from industrial sources into the air and approximately the same number are routinely sprayed on food crops as pesticides.

The incidence of breast cancer has increased considerably over the last fifty years, and some debates have centred on a possible link with environmental chemicals that mimic or disrupt the action of oestrogenic female hormones. The question is difficult to resolve, due to many uncertainties relating to the complexity of the disease. As in other malignancies, breast cancer is likely to arise when a breast tissue cell escapes the normal restraints on division and multiplies in an uncontrolled fashion. As detailed in the previous chapter, this requires the progressive accumulation of mutations in genes that control cell division and DNA maintenance. A further requirement is the specific promotion of the growth of such abnormal cells and, in the case of breast cancer, female sex hormones may play a role in this central process. Sustained, long-term exposure to the female hormone oestriol (an oestrogen) is a notable risk factor for breast cancer, for instance in women who have had early onset of menstruation or who have never breast-fed a child. This suggests that too much natural female sex hormone is hazardous. It has been suggested that synthetic chemicals that mimic the action of female sex hormones may be an additional risk factor.

Sex hormones are produced and released into the bloodstream from ovaries and testes. They constitute a group of chemical signal molecules that circulate in the bloodstream to coordinate the functions of various tissues and organs by interacting with specific target cells, thereby programming their activities. Each hormone, once it reaches a target cell, is taken inside, where it binds to a receptor protein. These receptors act as the initial, switch-like component in a set of events that can lead to activation of genes encoding proteins required, for example, for sexual development. The complex formed between the hormone and its receptor interacts with special DNA sequences that lie ahead of all the genes that the hormone is responsible for switching on. The appropriate tissue development then follows the switching on of these particular genes. Androgenic (male) hormones, such as *testosterone*, are involved in switching on genes for masculinization; oestrogenic (female) hormones, such as *oestrogen*, are responsible for the activation of genes that promote feminization. The sex hormones are also involved in switching on genes controlling reproductive functions in adult life such as the menstrual cycle and sperm production.

Although male and female sex hormones are made within our bodies, functioning as chemical messengers, there is a serious concern that certain synthetic (and natural) chemicals that can also act like sex hormones, or significantly affect the way in which natural sex hormones work, are now present in the environment. Although they have been called various names they can simply be referred to as *hormone mimics* or *hormone disrupters* (see Table 11.1). In the case of female hormone mimics, the ability to enter cells and bind to the receptors for natural female hormones is a relatively common phenomenon. Once bound, the mimics may act to jam the gene switching mechanism either permanently on or permanently off. This can result in the inappropriate activation, or lack of activation, of genes vital to some reproductive function. There are other chemicals that can block the receptors for male hormones, and yet others that can interfere with the circulation of natural sex hormones around the body.

From experiments with animals, it appears that exposure to some of these chemicals can alter sexual function and reproductive organs, or affect sexual development and function in the offspring of exposed pregnant mothers. Such chemicals get into the environment by a number of different routes. Although ostensibly reducing waste, incinerators are a significant source of atmospheric contamination. Amongst the pollutants released are dioxins. One of these, *TCCD*, can antagonize the effects of the female sex hormones. This harms normal sexual behaviour, sperm production and the reproductive capacity of male rats. The fungicide vinclozolin, which antagonizes the effect of male sex hormones, damages reproductive organs in male offspring when given to pregnant rats. Certain *phthalates* (used in the manufacture of plastic packaging for foods) reduce testosterone levels and shrink the testicles of male rats. In addition, PCBs (polychlorinated biphenyls) and dioxins, as well as thiocarbamide and sulphonamide pesticides, can act to disrupt the action of another group of our hormones produced by thyroid glands.

Before all synthetic chemicals are stigmatized, it should be pointed out that *hormone mimics are not all synthetic*. Some can be found in naturally occurring sources. For example, clover, a common fodder crop, is rich in naturally occurring compounds that can mimic the effects of female sex hormones. In general, environmental hormone mimics or disrupters are most likely to be ingested along with animal fats in the diet. Fatty foods from animals at the top of the food chain will contain the highest levels of these compounds, due to their progressive accumulation in the fatty tissues. In fairness, however, it should be made clear that, in many animal studies, where adverse effects were noted, the doses of mimics were far in excess of those likely to be found in food. Moreover, the amount of natural sex hormones to which most of us have been exposed in our normal lives is estimated to be millions of times greater than the amounts of synthetic mimics we are likely to encounter during our lifetime. Nevertheless, it should be emphasized that a reliable estimate of the total human exposure to natural and synthetic hormone mimics and disrupters is not yet available. Despite this, in terms of direct effects there is clear evidence of higher rates of reproductive abnormalities in the male and female children of mothers who took the drug diethylstilbestrol, which used to be prescribed to prevent miscarriages by acting as a hormone mimic.

**Table 11.1** Examples of chemical compounds with hormone mimic or disrupter activity

| Compound | Origin |
|---|---|
| DDT<br>Methoxychlor<br>Chlordecone<br>Atrazine | Organochlorine pesticides |
| Furans<br>Dioxins | Combustion and waste by-products |
| Alkylphenol polyethoxylates | Surfactants used in paints, pesticides and cleaning products, and as processing aids in paper and textile production |
| Bisphenol A | Breakdown product of polycarbonates used in resins for can linings and white dental fillings |
| Nonylphenol | Softener for plastics |
| Polychlorinated bipenyls (PCBs) | Electrical insulation |
| Phthalate esters | Plasticizers found in food packaging plastics |
| Vinclozolin | Fungicide |
| Phytoestrogens<br>(natural plant-derived<br>oestrogen mimics) | In clover, parsley, sage, garlic, wheat, oats, rye, barley, hops, rice, cabbage, soybean, potatoes, carrots, beans, apples, cherries, plums, pomegranates, coffee, whisky |

*Source*: Adapted from Burdon (1999).

Whereas natural female sex hormones are removed through normal metabolic pathways, such routes are usually not available to hormone mimics. Breast cancer patients have often been observed to have higher levels of DDE and PCBs in their tumours than in surrounding normal tissues. Although the possible role of PCBs and DDE in the development of human breast cancer remains a matter of speculation at present, experiments with rats and mice suggest that both have strong links with breast cancers that develop in these animals.

Many organochlorides that can function as hormone disrupters are highly persistent in air and water. In the case of one of these, DDT, seven years have to elapse before the levels in air or water are reduced to half their original level. Such organochlorides become deposited in the soil and on vegetation as a result of winds and storms. From there, they enter the food chain with the result that the diet is the main route of exposure. Although in most countries DDT and PCBs were banned in the 1970s, both can still be detected in human tissues. By 1951, DDT-contaminated breast milk was passing from mother to child. In tissues, DDT is converted to DDE, and an accumulation of DDE has been observed as we age, particularly in fatty tissues.

Animal studies have shown links between certain chemicals and cancers. In the wild, animals inhabiting contaminated environments have developed cancers; in the laboratory many synthetic (and natural) compounds will induce cancers in animals, particularly rodents. With the exception of the link between tobacco smoke and lung cancers, precise effects in humans have been more difficult to establish. At present tobacco smoke tops the lists of lethal carcinogens. It is believed to cause least a third of all cancers in the USA.

Cigarette smoking can cause a number of different cancers. Not only is it central to the generation of cancer of the lung, the respiratory tract, oesophagus, bladder and pancreas; it also probably causes cancers of the stomach, liver and kidney, as well as being implicated in chronic myelocytic leukaemia and colorectal cancer. Although the passive inhalation of environmental tobacco smoke causes less lung cancer than active smoking, as many as a few thousand deaths annually in the USA are attributable to second-hand smoke. Analyses of air samples from urban areas indicate that chronic exposure to high levels of air pollution can also increase lung cancer risk, particularly among those who already smoke. Diesel exhaust is likely to be a major hazard in this context, although sulphur dioxide from the burning of low-grade coal may also be significant.

Despite a lack of hard evidence, there is reason to suspect that *phenoxyherbicides* may be connected with non-Hodgkin's lymphoma, which has tripled in incidence since 1950. Multiple myeloma has also increased over this period, and may be associated with exposure to a variety of chemicals including metals, rubber, paints, solvents and petroleum products. Farmers and agricultural workers exposed to pesticides and herbicides also show a higher rate of this condition. In the case of bladder cancers, there is suspicion that exposure to aromatic amines such as aniline, benzidine, naphthylamine and toluidine, as well as cigarette smoking, may be critical. In the past, workers directly involved in dyestuffs or tyre production were most susceptible, but now these carcinogens are widely present in rivers, ground water and dump sites. The incidence of bladder cancer increased some 10 per cent in the USA between 1973 and 1991, although there is the possibility that half of these cases may be due to cigarette smoking. In the case of aromatic amines it is not all gloom; we do have some protection. Cells have proteins called *acetyl transferases* that can carry out the detoxification of aromatic amines (see Chapter 5). As was the case for the cytochrome P450s, the efficiency of the acetyl transferase proteins varies between individuals. Those who have inherited a poor level of acetyl transferase may thus be more at risk from bladder cancers caused by these aromatic amines.

## Evaluation of carcinogens

The process of cancer development is complex, and our ability to evaluate chemicals and other environmental factors in this context still requires a fuller understanding of all the different cellular mechanisms involved. In addition, because the process of development is usually quite lengthy, adequate testing of suspected carcinogens is fraught with technical difficulties. Many substances have been branded as human carcinogens merely on the basis of tests carried out in experimental animals (usually rodents) over very short time periods, often with inappropriately high concentrations of the chemical in question. Whilst providing useful indicators of potential carcinogenicity, such animal tests fail abysmally to provide the necessary hard information regarding the real dangers to humans faced with long-term, low-level exposures to hazardous substances, which also may accumulate to different extents in different cells and tissues. Although this can be partly a function of their different rates of breakdown in varying tissues, a further concern is that the products of their breakdown could be even more carcinogenic. The possibility that substances which are carcinogenic in rodents may simply not be carcinogenic for humans and vice versa makes the situation even more complex and potentially misleading. Moreover, potentially adverse effects may be ameliorated by differences in the effectiveness of the detoxifying systems that we have inherited. On top of all this is the complex problem of simulating environmental reality. In most situations, we are not exposed to a single carcinogen at a time. But this is all that most present toxicity tests can adequately deal with. Over long periods of time we may be exposed to veritable cocktails of environmental carcinogens, some with the propensity to accumulate in certain of our tissues, but not in others. Some may also have the ability to act in concert with others to potentiate their harmful effects, and some may be converted within our bodies to an unknown variety of potentially even more carcinogenic substances. Finally, there is the additional complexity that carcinogens can act in different ways. As will be recalled, some act as initiators and mutate DNA, but others can function to promote the growth of tumour precursor cells.

On the face of it, there is a pressing need for a more rigorous evaluation and awareness of the increasing hazards of synthetic chemicals in the environment. Much has already been done to protect those in the workplace with appropriate legislation, but there are insufficient safeguards for the public at large. The issues involved are undoubtedly complex, but too often the acquisition of the relevant knowledge has been slow. There is a sharp contrast between the very conservative attitude, at least in Scotland, towards problems with mobile phones (see Chapter 4), and the somewhat laissez-faire approach to potentially hazardous chemicals. By the time the real hazards of a particular environmental chemical are understood, the process of cancer development in afflicted victims is usually well advanced. It not surprising that the possibilities of having drugs available that might provide instant cures for cancers in advanced states is a very attractive dream for these victims.

Although it could be argued that cancers are likely to have little effect on our future evolution, since they mainly affect individuals past their reproductive age, chemicals that can cause mutations in sperm or eggs may well be more significant, although in no readily predictable way. Those chemicals, such as hormone mimics, which can cause reproductive problems undoubtedly have more ominous implications for our continued survival.

For many synthetic carcinogens, eradication from the environment can only be a very long-term target. It is not a simple matter to avoid many of them, as it is currently to evade exposure to tobacco smoke. Some protective strategies have been suggested which involve the development of new drugs for *chemointervention*. The aim is to use novel drugs to induce increased levels of the detoxifying proteins within cells, in an attempt to neutralize environmental carcinogens before they can do their damage to DNA. However, considering the long-term nature of the carcinogenic process, these protective drugs would inevitably have to be taken on a prolonged basis, with the attendant risk of undesirable side effects.

## Are we digging our own graves with our knives and forks?

It has been suggested that the proportion of cancer deaths due to diet in the USA may be equivalent to that caused by tobacco smoke. What is clear is that many potential carcinogens now contaminate drinking water, and are routinely sprayed on food crops as pesticides. One recent commentator has even suggested that we are 'digging our own graves with our knives and forks'.

In general, foodstuffs contain many thousands of different chemicals, both natural and synthetic, and it is difficult to be specific with regard to all possible carcinogens. Despite this (as pointed out in Chapter 6) food components such as aflatoxins, from contaminating moulds, do cause liver cancers in humans. In general, however, although foodstuffs and beverages contain large numbers of compounds, the ability of some of these to cause cancers has only been demonstrated in laboratory animals, and only at concentrations vastly in excess of what might normally be encountered in the human diet.

Closer inspection of the possible connections between cancer deaths and diet has indicated that the problem is not necessarily what is present in the diet, but rather what is missing. For instance, diets that are deficient in fruits and vegetables can considerably increase the risks of certain cancers. Epidemiologists have demonstrated impressive protection by diets rich in fruits and vegetables against cancers of the lung, oral cavity, larynx, oesophagus, stomach, pancreas, cervix, colon, rectum, ovary and bladder. Those in the population with the lowest intake of fruits and vegetables have almost double the normal incidence of these cancers. For breast and prostate cancers the figures are, however, less impressive. Possible explanations of the protective effects brought about by high dietary intakes of fruit and vegetables (four to five helpings a day) are complex. There are compounds naturally present in plants that can significantly increase the activity of cellular detoxifying proteins and thus help to neutralize environmental carcinogens before they can do their damage to DNA. Examples are the allyl sulphides present in garlic and onions; the dithiolthiones and isothiocyanates in cruciferous vegetables such as broccoli, cabbage and cauliflower; quercitin in apples and onions; and ellagic acid in strawberries, raspberries, blackberries, walnuts and pecans. Fruits and vegetables also contain many substances capable of acting as antioxidants such as tocopherols, carotenoids and flavonoids (see Chapter 9). At present these is an increasing interest in the protective role of dietary vitamin E, vitamin C and beta-carotene in lowering the incidence of a range of human tumours. In general, these plant-derived antioxidants could diminish the opportunity for reactive free radicals, derived from external environmental sources or from within cells, to damage DNA.

Despite the extremely convincing epidemiological evidence of preventative anti-cancer strategies involving dietary fruits and vegetables, it has been argued that these simultaneously carry the risks of synthetic pesticide contamination. Fruits and vegetables, of course, already contain high levels of *natural* pesticides. They make these in an attempt to protect themselves, as much as possible, from fungal invasion, as well as attack by predators such as insects and herbivorous animals. Unlike man, plants cannot run away and hide from such dangers. Compared with the level of these natural plant pesticides, contamination with synthetic pesticides is usually extremely small. Nonetheless, it should be stressed that the synthetic pesticides are contaminants and do not actually belong naturally in plant-derived foodstuffs. The recent popularity of organically grown fruits and vegetables may well reduce the level of contamination with synthetic pesticides, but this may be at the cost of failing to eliminate the contamination of crop plants with various fungal infestations. In turn, these may present different haz-ards, such as the presence of fungal toxins, akin to the cancer-causing aflatoxins. Of course, organically grown fruit and vegetables probably contain the same amounts of natural pesticides as those grown by other farming methods.

## Can radiation be safe?

In the early 1930s, the experiments of Hermann Muller with fruit flies very clearly indicated that X-rays were powerful agents of mutation, and many early workers with X-rays subsequently died of cancer. We now know that ionizing radiation can cause damage to components of DNA, as well as being responsible for single- and double-strand break-ages. While we can usually repair DNA single-strand breaks fairly efficiently, other types of DNA damage are more persistent and can cause mutations and even cell death, if the damage is severe. Attempts by our repair systems to rectify double-strand breaks can sometimes lead to disastrous results. Quite large segments of DNA can become duplicated, deleted, reversed or repositioned. After the nuclear acci-dent at the Chernobyl reactor in the Ukraine in April 1986, where many individuals were heavily exposed to radiation, there was evidence for DNA rearrangements in some victims, as well as increases in the incidence of thyroid cancer in children. Moreover, studies carried out on the population as far as 200 km to the north revealed a doubling of the mutation rate in their somatic cells, even ten years on.

As described in Chapter 3, the progressive irradiation of our planet began following World War II. At that time, the superpowers vied with one another to construct bigger and better nuclear weapons, and to make their advances clear to their opponents by demonstrations, in an orgy of open-air testing. Between 1952 and 1963, radioactive fall-out became extensively distributed over the earth's surface as a result of winds and rainfall. Some twenty years later, rates of childhood cancers and leukaemia began to rise. By 1970, most of us had plutonium and strontium from atmospheric fallout in our bodies, and whilst nuclear testing, thankfully, was phased out in the 1960s, the hazards from radioactivity did not diminish. Controlled and accidental releases from nuclear power stations and reprocessing plants replaced bombs. Accidents involving nuclear reactors are still a daily possibility and must be considered to be a potentially regular feature of the nuclear age.

Despite our considerable accumulation of knowledge, it is still difficult to decide what is a safe dose of radioactivity. Moreover, the appearance of cancers is not proportional to the dose. Cells that are actually in the process of dividing are extremely sensitive to radiation, whereas cells that normally divide rarely, and constitute the majority in our bodies, are relatively immune. Thus, quite low radiation doses can damage DNA in dividing cells, thereby causing mutations and increasing the rate of cancer development. At higher radiation doses, cell death predominates over mutation and the cancer incidence drops. Among the survivors of the Japanese cities blasted by atomic bombs in 1945, and thus exposed to high levels of radiation, only 1 per cent died of cancers related to ionizing radiation. The large dose of radiation that they undoubtedly received was, however, only a single dose and largely external. This contrasts with situations in which radioactive substances, such as strontium 90, are inhaled or ingested (as already described in Chapter 3), and serve as long-term internal sources of radiation. Strontium 90 can concentrate in tissues like bone and also in chromosomes, where it replaces the naturally occurring calcium atoms. Particles of radioactive dust can also enter the body by ingestion or by inhalation into the lungs, and through the lungs into the lymphatic system, where they can coat membrane surfaces and cause massive irradiation to surrounding cells and tissues. A particle containing plutonium 239 trapped in a lymph node can emit alpha particles essentially on a continuous basis.

When around 31,000 descendants of the survivors of the Japanese atomic blasts were studied, relatively little evidence of extensive hereditary effects turned up. This dearth of extra mutations, cancers or inherited diseases in later generations is quite surprising and difficult to explain. It may be that the DNA of human eggs and sperm is in some way shielded from the effects of external radiation. Alternatively, these germ cells may have extremely efficient DNA repair mechanisms, or mechanisms for programmed cell death in the face of hopelessly damaged DNA, which are readily triggered. Despite this important statistic, there are still suggestions that the children of men exposed to radiation at work, for example at nuclear power stations or reprocessing plants, have a higher than normal risk of developing leukaemia. Investigations so far indicate that this risk is not directly related to the external radiation dose suffered by the fathers. Although it is difficult to measure, it may be important in this case to consider the possibility of internal radiation effects, for instance from ingested or inhaled radioactive substances or particles.

Despite the very real concerns regarding the safety of the nuclear industry, it is important to see them in a wider context. At the present time, only about 2 per cent of cancer deaths in the USA can be specifically ascribed to any type of radiation. Putting this into some perspective, the number of such deaths is equivalent to a mere 6 per cent of the cancer deaths due to cigarette smoking. Of these radiation cancers, the major proportion are attributable to skin cancers caused by ultraviolet rays from the sun, which, in principle, can be avoided. As we have seen (Chapter 8), three forms of skin cancer are observed: squamous cell carcinomas, basal cell carcinomas and melanomas. The last of these is relatively uncommon, representing only about 4 per cent of annual skin cancer cases in the USA. Studies of squamous skin cell carcinomas, which occur especially on the faces and hands of whites living in the tropics, indicate mutations at particular sites in the tumour suppressor gene encoding the important protein p53. The same has been observed for basal skin carcinomas, but not for melanomas. Dermatologists have recognized that, when skin becomes sunburned, some cells undergo apoptosis (programmed cell death) (see Chapter 10). In general, it seems that apoptosis is important in the prevention of non-melanoma skin cancers. Loss of p53 function may prevent skin cells from initiating this programmed death process in the face of high levels of UV-initiated DNA damage. In contrast, the mechanisms involved in the triggering of melanoma are not yet understood.

Other sources of radiation such as electric power lines, household appliances and cellular phones do not contribute significantly to the cancer death statistics at present and diagnostic X-rays yield compensatory benefits. Even the risks of radon, which has been linked to lung cancer, are now reduced by recent improvements in the ventilation of buildings.

## Can we minimize the risks of cancer from environmental carcinogens?

A reasonable strategy for reducing the risks of cancer would be simply to try to steer clear of known carcinogens in the environment and workplace, eat plenty of fruit and vegetables, stay out of intense sunlight and avoid tobacco smoke, automobile exhaust fumes and nuclear radiation. There is, however, now speculation that more insidious risks exist from hormonal mimics, or disrupters, which may be linked with hormone-related cancers such as breast, ovarian and cervical cancers in women and prostate and testicular cancers in men. Some hormone mimics find their way into our environment as pesticides, as insulators, as processing aids in paper and textile production, as components of plastics and paints, and through combustion and waste by-products (for a detailed listing, see Table 11.1). Although there is a pressing requirement for more solid evidence, it might be considered prudent to limit the intake of foods that have at some time been exposed to plastics (especially fatty foods which absorb such compounds more easily). This is not as easy at it seems. Plastic food packaging is now used for a major proportion of our foods, but this is not always obvious. For example, there is usually a thin layer of plastic coating the inside of the cartons and cans used for most drinks. A switch to mineral water bottled in glass rather than plastic, and the limitation of food wrapped in plastic films are other possibilities. Unfortunately, a satisfactory evaluation of the risks relating to environmental hormone mimics and disrupters is likely to be a long time in coming. There are still many uncertainties regarding the development of the hormone-related cancers, thus making it difficult to place mimics and disrupters in a meaningful scientific context, and to assess what levels in our diet may pose real threats. This does not mean we should just ignore them. We should be aware of the potential risks.

## Is personal risk assessment a possibility?

Because the timescale of cancer development is so long, it might be nice to imagine that, well before any tumour became a problem, we could visit a laboratory that would assess our tissues for biological clues, or *biomarkers*, that would indicate the extent of our own personal risk. The assessment, involving suitable biomarkers, would aim to determine the extent to which we had already been assaulted by cancer-causing agents, and take account of our likely personal special vulnerability to the effects of carcinogens in the environment. These would obviously include tobacco smoke, radiation, natural and synthetic chemicals in food, water and air, and so on. Discovery of suitable biomarkers might well help affected individuals to prevent cancer, as they would at least know what carcinogens they most needed to avoid. It would also pinpoint where there was increased risk in certain groups of the population, and trigger public health services to take new steps to reduce exposures that are beyond the ability of any one individual to control. It could also assist in forward-planning procedures for cancer treatment.

What biomarkers suggest an increased cancer risk? By the 1980s it was known that a well-established group of carcinogens, namely the polycyclic aromatic hydrocarbons (PAHs), left a readily recognizable fingerprint in human lung and liver cells. This takes the form of a quite bulky modification to certain nucleotides of the DNA within these cells. This particular modification is often referred to as a *PAH-adduct*. Soon it was possible to show that people known to have been exposed to high levels of PAHs from tobacco smoke, polluted air or certain industrial sites had a higher than normal number of PAH-adducts in the DNA isolated from their blood cells. The possible use of such a measurement as a biomarker of heightened cancer risk was supported by the observation that cells with higher than normal levels of PAH-adducts also exhibited higher than normal levels of mutations and chromosomal abnormalities common in tumour cells. Whether or not the presence of abnormal levels of PAH-adducts will be able to predict lung cancer well in advance of symptoms and/or clinical diagnosis remains to be seen.

Other potential biomarkers suggest themselves. With regard to exposure to carcinogens, DNA could be isolated from tissues to determine whether it had been modified, for example by aflatoxins from the diet. The extent of free radical damage to DNA could also be assessed by measuring the level of a particular modified nucleotide component called *8-hydroxy guanine*, which is a well-known unique fingerprint of free radical damage. Having isolated some tissue DNA, it is also possible to use it to assess the amount and location of all mutations in the gene that encodes the key controlling protein, p53. Mutations in this gene are already known to increase the risk for a number of cancers, as discussed earlier. The precise pattern of damage to the p53 gene will also provide clues as to what particular carcinogen has been responsible.

These biomarkers assess our history of exposure to carcinogens. Another type of biomarker to pursue is one that will indicate inherited susceptibility to cancer. It is possible to take blood cell samples and determine the range of cytochrome P450 proteins that an individual has inherited, together with an indication of their overall detoxification capabilities of these proteins in detoxifying environmental chemicals. The same, of course, could be done for an individual's glutathione transferases and acetyl transferases, which also detoxify environmental chemicals, but in different ways. People vary in their responses to carcinogens because they inherit different forms of these detoxifying proteins. The particular forms that one person inherits may be more, or less helpful, than those another person possesses. At the same time as these tests are being carried out, DNA could also be isolated from the blood cell sample and tested for occurrence of mutations that would indicate an inherited susceptibility to cancers. In this context it would be particularly useful to screen tumour suppressor genes, such as those encoding the retinoblastoma protein and the p53 protein (see Chapter 10). Examination of the gene BRCA1 for mutations will also indicate increased risk of breast cancer (see also Chapter 10). Yet other types of potentially useful biomarkers would be the concentrations in blood of food-derived antioxidants, as well as vitamins C and E. These would indicate whether the individual had a good chance of dealing with any excesses of free radicals that might be potentially damaging to their DNA.

Clearly it is possible to expand this list of potential biomarkers of risk on a continuous basis as our knowledge of cancer and its origins becomes more extensive. A basic objective is to improve estimates of cancer risk by analysing variations in the innate and acquired susceptibility within human populations. It is hoped that determination of multiple traits, combined with biological assessment of exposure and early damage, will, in time, yield more precise and meaningful estimates of personal risk. All of this seems quite laudable, but one difficulty might well be that those participating in this type of screening may need to be wary of potential prejudice from insurance companies. On a more positive note, risk assessment may reduce the hazardous behaviour of individuals. For example, people found to be significantly at risk might opt to improve their diets or stop smoking. Risk assessment might also force legislative bodies to limit involuntary exposure to carcinogenic substances in air, water, food and the workplace. It has been suggested that, in the absence of all environmental exposures, the occurrence of cancers might be diminished by as much as a staggering 90 per cent. Prevention is the best cure!

## Fighting cancer with therapeutic drugs that attack DNA

Sometimes it is simply too late to assess personal risk and take avoiding action. By the time the hazards of a particular chemical are clearly understood, the process of tumour development in those exposed some years previously may be well advanced. Not surprisingly, this drives the quest for effective anticancer drugs for victims with advanced cancers. *Chemotherapy* involving drugs is a common approach to cancer treatment. Paradoxically, many presently used cancer treatments depend on the use of therapeutic drugs capable of attacking DNA. Moreover, these are often combined with radiotherapy, which, as was outlined in Chapter 3, capitalizes on the ability of strong ionizing radiation to kill cells by severely damaging DNA.

Curiously, the starting point for the development of some successful anticancer drugs was the study of some extremely toxic synthetic chemicals that were originally created for release into the environment as chemical weapons. World War I saw the first serious use of chemicals as weapons of mass destruction. Poison gases killed or wounded one and a half million people. Thousands more died from their effects after 1918, and chemical warfare came to be regarded with particular revulsion. Yet, despite attempts to outlaw them, chemical weapons have continued to be developed and even used. The Italians and the Japanese used mustard gas in the 1930s and the Nazis developed deadly nerve gases in 1937, building up a huge arsenal of chemical weaponry that Hitler came close to using on several occasions during World War II. In more recent times, there is strong evidence to suggest that the Russians in their invasion of Afghanistan (1980–96) deployed chemical weapons. Today, as well as being a direct threat to human life, chemical weapons remain a serious environmental threat in the wrong hands.

Mustard gas, a highly toxic alkyl halide, was used extensively in World War I and stockpiled by many nations as a deterrent, until several international treaties in the 1980s banned its use and sought the destruction of existing stocks. When this gas makes contact with the lungs it causes extensive blistering, tissue destruction and death, if the exposure is severe. Some twenty-five years later, during World War II, a group of tertiary amines called *nitrogen mustards*, with properties quite similar to mustard gas, were investigated intensively as alternative chemical warfare agents. One interesting property of these highly toxic chemicals is their ability, when absorbed into cells, to straddle the two strands that make up DNA molecules, and chemically link them together effectively forming an 'interstrand cross-link'. This would prevent the separation of the two strands during the process of chromosome replication (see Chapter 5).

Because of their potential ability to interfere with the vital process of chromosome replication and gene action, studies were initiated in the USA in 1942 to evaluate the clinical potential of nitrogen mustards to block the division of cancer cells. As will be recalled from earlier chapters, cancer cells gain the ability to divide uncontrollably, so chemicals that could interfere with cell division by targeting the DNA copying phase were seen to offer therapeutic possibilities. Initially, using experimental animals, it was found that the damage done after nitrogen mustard was absorbed through the skin was of greater consequence than the initial blistering action on the skin. The toxicity was most extensive towards cells in the animal that normally divided rapidly, such as the cells in lymphoid tissue and bone marrow. In this respect, these preliminary studies confirmed the suspicion that the mustards could interfere with cell division processes, and suggested that they might be effective against the uncontrolled division of cancer cells. With this in mind, nitrogen mustards were then tested against lymphomas (lymphoid cancers) in experimental animals, with remarkable success in terms of remissions and/or prolongation of life. By late 1942, the first human trial was under way. Although the patient was apparently in a hopeless situation, suffering a lymphoma that was not responding to radiation treatment, a course of treatment with a nitrogen mustard codenamed HN3 led to a notable improvement even by the second day, although there were signs of damage to normal bone marrow cells brought about by the drug. Nevertheless, after two weeks there were no signs of the tumour. However, the next few weeks saw not only the regeneration of the bone marrow cells but also re-emergence of the cancer. A year later, use of another nitrogen mustard, HN2 (later called mustine), produced spectacular remissions in patients with Hodgkin's disease. By 1946, it was clear that HN2 and HN3 could produce useful results in patients with Hodgkin's disease, lymphomas and chronic leukaemia. In contrast, they were less effective against acute leukaemia and other types of cancer. These pioneering studies involving an alternative use of chemical warfare agents set the scene for a dramatic post-war expansion in the development of cancer chemotherapeutic drugs, many of which, rather than aiming to kill cancer cells directly, sought to interfere with the processes of DNA copying and thereby block cancer cell replication. Although the initial development of nitrogen mustards for cancer chemotherapy took place some sixty years ago, one, mechlorethamine, is still in use today. Another synthetic chemical related to nitrogen mustards, and also developed to cross-link DNA strands, is the drug cyclophosphamide, which still remains useful against a wide range of tumours. More recent examples of cross-linking anticancer drugs are mitomycin C, used in the treatment of gastrointestinal and bladder cancers, and cisplatin, which is often used against cancers of the ovary.

*Acridine dyes* are another group of hazardous synthetic environmental chemicals capable of damaging DNA. These dyestuffs cause problems because their molecules can squeeze themselves into the space between individual nucleotides of DNA molecules. This is called *intercalation* and, as might be expected, distorts the normal structure of the afflicted DNA molecules so that their copying is impaired, as is the decoding of their genes. The ability to intercalate into DNA has, nevertheless, been the basis for the action of a range of novel anticancer drugs created naturally by various microbes including daunorubicin, doxorubicin and actinomycin D. The last of these has been particularly useful in the fight against testicular cancers and Wilm's tumour in children. Doxorubicin, despite showing some toxicity towards the heart, is of considerable value in the treatment of acute leukaemias, lymphomas (non-Hodgkin's) and many solid tumours.

*Psoralens* comprise another group of synthetic chemicals, developed to intercalate between DNA nucleotides. However, to be effective, these drugs have to anchored in place within the target DNA molecules. In practice, this is achieved by irradiation with long-wave ultraviolet light. Such an ultraviolet-induced linkage with DNA prevents subsequent chromosome replication and has facilitated the use of psoralens in the treatment of psoriasis, a condition characterized by excessive production of skin cells. Following application of the psoralens to the afflicted skin tissues, it is particularly easy in dermatology clinics to carry out their fixation to skin cell DNA by focusing some ultraviolet light at the psoralen-treated skin area. A word of caution, however, since psoralens also occur naturally in foodstuffs such as parsley, parsnips and celery. If taken in excessive quantities, there is a worry that such vegetables could be an unwelcome source of psoralens, potentially damaging to DNA molecules, especially in our tissues that might be exposed to excessive levels of ultraviolet radiation from sunlight or ultraviolet lamps. Unfortunately, at present there are no clear indications of what might constitute a hazardous dose of such dietary psoralens.

Besides therapeutic drugs that attack the DNA of tumour cells, ionizing radiation, which can severely damage DNA, has also been used in cancer therapy. However, like the drugs, there is the problem of incomplete specificity. In addition to suppressing the propagation of tumour cells, the division of other cells of the body such as intestinal cells and bone marrow cells can also be affected. This has stimulated many other approaches to cancer treatment that do not involve attack on DNA. However, in no case is there yet a drug, or treatment, that is guaranteed to provide a permanent cure for cancer. Prevention therefore still tops the list as the best cure.

**Key points in this chapter**

- Epidemiologists seek to evaluate the environmental causes of various cancers. They identify factors that are common to cancer victims and evaluate them in the context of current biological and medical knowledge.
- There are many difficulties that prevent the truly meaningful risk assessment of environmental carcinogens.
- Our diet contains many thousands of different chemicals, some natural and others present as environmental pollutants. The aflatoxins, arising from fungal contaminations, are established carcinogens. From the health point of view, the problem is more often what is not in our diet. Diets deficient in fruits and vegetables can increase the risks of certain cancers.
- The increasing incidence of breast cancer has raised questions regarding the role and occurrence of environmental chemicals that mimic female sex hormones.
- Despite considerable knowledge of the DNA-damaging capabilities of ionizing radiation, it is still difficult to decide what is a safe dose of radioactivity.
- There are definite steps that we can take to minimize the risks of cancer from environmental carcinogens. Soon, personal risk assessment will be a possibility.
- If cancer develops, it is possible to attempt to fight the disease with various drugs and radiotherapy. Some of the therapeutic drugs used are, paradoxically, based on their ability to attack DNA. As yet there is no drug, or treatment, that provides a truly permanent cure.
- Cancer prevention still remains the best cure.

# Could gene damage redirect our evolution?

The word 'mutation' may conjure up visions of grotesque, humanoid monsters. On top of this, the idea that environmental factors can cause a significant number of mutations could well kindle fears that some sort of apocalypse is nigh, given the worrying changes in our current environment. It is quite understandable to ask whether these environmental changes will endanger not only our present health and lifestyle but also the way in which humankind might evolve in the future. The possibility that the environment could influence evolution certainly exercised the minds of a number of eminent biologists in the nineteenth century. Some believed that characteristics acquired during one's lifetime could be passed on to future generations. For example, if you had an accident during childhood in which you lost a toe, then there was a probability that your children might be born with a toe missing. Jean Baptiste Lamarck, one of the great French biologists of the nineteenth century, took the view that children inherited the characteristics acquired during the life of their parents. Not only did he believe that living things inherited acquired characteristics, he also thought that such variability in the characteristics was tuned to the organism's particular requirements. For instance, if an animal such as a giraffe found its environment deficient in easily accessible vegetation, it might have to stretch its neck to reach a meal of leaves in higher locations. Gradually, over a number of generations, the animal's neck would become progressively elongated to satisfy this necessity. Such events, in Lamarck's view, accounted for the evolution of giraffes in relation to their environment. For humans, the idea that acquired characteristics could be inherited might understandably promote specifically focused parental behaviour. If a strong baby was desired, one might expect to see prospective parents in the gymnasium on daily weight-lifting programmes. For a more intelligent baby, it might be necessary for intending parents to hone their general knowledge skills and abilities at mental arithmetic, and so on. Despite the naivety of these ideas, they may have a superficial attractiveness for some. However, no firm evidence has ever been produced to suggest that acquired characteristics can be inherited. Indeed, in 1904 a German zoologist August Weissmann carried out a convincing test to the contrary. He cut off the tails from male and female mice before permitting them to mate. He then took the progeny that resulted and repeated the process over a further twenty-two generations. The bottom line was that none of the offspring that emerged from any of these generations had tails any shorter than those of normal mice. The major problem with Lamarck's theory was simply that it was wrong. Indeed, modern knowledge of genetics and DNA makes his views appear somewhat ludicrous. Lamarck, of course, did not have the benefit of such knowledge.

## Natural selection

Throughout most of our history we have taken our planet very much for granted, but by the nineteenth century Victorian society had developed a grand passion for natural history or the study of nature. Myriads of plant and animal species were avidly collected and catalogued by enthusiastic amateurs pursuing biology as an innocent hobby. Fossils were hunted out in enormous numbers and a greater understanding of the earth's geology emerged.

Among the dedicated amateurs of the time was Charles Darwin, who had already considered careers both in the Church and in medicine. In 1831, at the age of 22, he sailed out of Plymouth, as a naturalist, on a now famous circumnavigation of the world aboard the HMS *Beagle*. After five years he returned home to England, his head full of ideas that would later change for ever views on evolutionary history and religion. Darwin followed the tradition of the time for patient collecting and painstaking observation of animals and plants.

During the long voyage he developed into an excellent naturalist, constantly observing and thinking about the plethora of geological and biological phenomena that confronted him. It was his interpretations that were to shake the conventional wisdom of the time. After his return in 1836 he never left England again and spent the rest of his years in the countryside with his wife and family. By 1837 Darwin had significant doubts that species were permanent and unchangeable and, although he was occupied between then and 1859 with many various scientific activities, the question of the origin of species was never far from his thoughts. During these years he read widely and experimented carefully, and came to the view that it was *natural selection* that decides which animal or plant survives and is fit to breed. His observations also suggested that naked competition and blind chance have dictated our origins. Despite his twenty-year search for conclusive evidence, Darwin was so conscious of many gaps in his thesis that he might never have made his views public. Although many biologists had recognized some variation within species, those before Darwin maintained that the extent of any variation was strictly limited. In 1858, another naturalist, Alfred Russell Wallace, then working in the Far East, arrived at remarkably similar views on the principles of natural selection. Communication between them finally spurred Darwin into formally publishing his own theories, although Wallace always gave Darwin credit for being first to discover natural selection. In 1859, Darwin's seminal book *On the Origin of Species by Means of Natural Selection* was eventually published. This event almost immediately transformed him into a public figure, vehemently denounced by the religious establishment of the time. Many fellow scientists were sceptical and initially opposed to Darwin's views. However, most were gradually won over, and by old age Darwin was widely respected. When Darwin died in 1882, he was buried in Westminster Abbey, although he received no official honour from the state during his life, such was the power of the religious establishment. Indeed, pockets of antagonism and denial still linger. As lately as 1997, the State Board of Education in Illinois, USA, did not permit any mention of evolution in its new state-wide standards, and the state of Kansas removed the term 'evolution' from its school science programmes.

## Evolution and the environment

While environmental factors can certainly cause mutations and influence the action of genes, it is nonetheless clear that the environment cannot direct evolution in any predictable way. Alterations to parts of an animal are not transmitted to its progeny, as was supposed by Lamarck and others. Rather, it is alterations, or mutations, in DNA that are passed from one generation to the next. A new characteristic can be inherited only if it results from an alteration in the DNA of eggs or sperm that is subsequently copied at each generation.

The particular contribution that Darwin made was to state that species were not specially created in their present form, but that they evolved from ancestral species by a mechanism that he called natural selection. At a general level, the theory of natural selection requires that individuals within a species vary from one another and that a considerable proportion of this variation is inherited. Moreover, organisms should have an ability to produce more progeny than the environment can support, so that, unavoidably, some will not survive. In this way only a proportion of the population will live and reproduce. Selection will favour those that are best adapted to their environment: for example, those that are best at locating food, or those better able to avoid being the meal of some predator, or those more able to tolerate the climatic conditions. Since much of the variation between individuals is inherited, those that can surmount these challenges and actually reproduce will pass on some of their attributes to their offspring. In short, the attributes that benefited an individual organism's survival and reproduction in certain specific environmental conditions tend to be the characteristics passed on to the next generation. When this is reiterated over many generations, organisms will evolve to possess attributes that favour their survival and reproduction in the prevailing environmental conditions, over less well adapted organisms. Although organisms are naturally selected to fit the prevailing environmental conditions, should these conditions change, then other variants in the population, better able to survive and reproduce, will progressively become dominant. In summary, evolutionary change is based mainly on interactions between populations of organisms and their environments. Evolution does not 'aim' to create an ideal species. It is about adaptation and survival and not about progression to some state of perfection. The fossil record is full of species that appeared to be strong and numerous, but that died off because they were simply unable to adapt to changing environmental circumstances.

Darwin's theory of natural selection has had many scientific and religious opponents over the years. These included the USSR, where it was criticized in sinister political terms, particularly by the favoured protégé of Stalin, Trofim Lysenko. He said that the theory of natural selection, along with Gregor Mendel's fundamental laws of heredity, had many capitalist overtones. What followed during the 1930s up to the mid-1960s within orthodox scientific circles of the USSR was little less than an an unprecedented reign of terror. Lysenko, a bogus geneticist and agricultural charlatan, demanded that all genetic research in the Soviet Union should conform to Marxist theory. In practice, this meant the acceptance of the discredited concepts of Lamarck regarding the inheritance of acquired characteristics. As a result, hundreds of the best Soviet biologists were dismissed, or demoted, for failing to go along with these fraudulent views. Lysenko bewitched Stalin with various apparently miraculous schemes, all purporting to bring about dramatic, short-term increases in food productivity with minimal financial outlay. Extensively promoted in the agricultural heartland, the plans failed abysmally, wasting millions of roubles. One example was his scheme to boost wheat production through 'vernalization', which he believed could be inherited. He proposed that winter varieties of cereals could be genetically converted to spring or summer varieties by cold treatment. We know now that none of the genes involved was altered in any way by the low-temperature treatment. Instead, the prior cold treatment merely substituted for the natural chilling period of winter, which is a necessary physiological requirement for growth and flowering of winter varieties in the following spring. Although Lysenko was never able to demonstrate the viability of his miracle claims by any reproducible experiments, it is believed that this is one reason why his assertions appealed to Stalin. They simply transcended the capitalist laws and theories of biological science, and little was done to deny that some of the marvels stemmed from the great Stalin himself. Rather than reinforcing Lamarck's views on the passing on of acquired characteristics, Lysenko's experiments merely lent weight to the opposition.

## Mutation and evolution

In situations where a gene harbours a mutation, this can affect the production of the protein it encodes. Many mutations can result in seriously flawed protein products, no longer able to carry out their normal role within cells. When considering the long-term effects of mutations, a key consideration relates to the cell type in which the DNA is afflicted. Exposure to the sun's ultraviolet radiation is more likely to cause mutations in the DNA of skin cells, rather than in the DNA of testes or ovary cells. These latter cells are simply more likely to be shielded from the sun. In contrast, cells of our ovaries or testes would be more vulnerable to the powerful penetrating power of X-rays or other forms of nuclear radiation. Inhalation, or ingestion, of many environmental pollutants would also result in their distribution to a wide variety of cells. Should mutations be induced in the DNA of sperm, or eggs, then the offspring that result following fertilization will inherit these mutations. In contrast, this would not be the case for mutations inflicted on the DNA of cells other than sperm or eggs. These other cells are the somatic cells; because they do not participate in the fertilization processes, mutations within their DNA cannot be passed on to future generations. This does not mean that mutations in somatic cells are of no consequence. Although ultraviolet radiation, for instance, is capable of inducing mutations in skin cells which will not be passed on to our children, these mutations can be passed on to other cells in skin. Normally skin is in a constant state of renewal. Dead skin cells slough off from the surface and are replaced by the division of younger skin cells lying underneath. In this way, a mutation can spread through groups of skin cells. However, like all mutations in somatic cells, they cease to exist when the individual dies. A problem only arises if the particular mutation that is being spread by this route is central to the development of skin cancers. A prime example would be a mutation occurring in the tumour suppressor gene that encodes the protein p53 (see Chapter 8).

Returning to the issue of sexual reproduction involving the sperm and eggs of our parents, we each inherit any mutations that our parents have inherited, together with any that had been inflicted on their sperm or egg cell DNA during the course of their lives prior to reproduction (estimates indicate that this could be approximately one or two mutations). On top of this, the genetic processes occurring in testes and ovaries, which lead to the creation of sperm and egg cells, themselves cause the rearrangement of some genes into fresh combinations. All of this means that we each finish up with a unique collection of mutations in our DNA. This is reflected in the individual variation that we can readily observe in human populations: for example, people look very different from one another and behave in quite distinct ways. Other variations, however, can escape notice because they can be extremely subtle. Nonetheless, it is these slight differences between individuals in a population of organisms that serve as the raw material for the process of natural selection originally proposed by Darwin. Genetic diversity is often taken as a sign of a healthy population, and the opportunities for genetic intermixing have increased in modern times. By contrast, in the Middle Ages people were able to travel only very short distances from their homes, which put severe constraints on their choice of sexual partner. Genetic inbreeding brings with it risks to health and fertility. We may prefer inbred pets and livestock because they may have more pleasing, or standardized, characteristics, but, in the long run, they are more vulnerable to diseases and other afflictions. In the agricultural world, commercial pressures have promoted the inbreeding of staple crops that are now more genetically uniform across the world. In the process, however, such crops may have lost the ability to resist various fungal infections or other stresses. Inbreeding can leave a plant or animal population vulnerable, especially if it is small or isolated.

## Survival and reproductive success

How exactly might mutations affect survival and reproductive success? This is a complex business, and is further complicated by the multiplicity of interactions between genes and their protein products, as well as the overall physiology of the organism. Despite these difficulties, we do know that some mutations have no effect one way or another on survival or reproduction. In other cases, the reproductive success of the afflicted organism may be seriously impaired, or, at the very least, the organism will find itself at a considerable competitive disadvantage. Genes that are ideal for one particular environment can be severely disadvantageous for another. Cattle bred for maximum milk or beef production in the temperate climes of the UK may quickly succumb if transported to tropical areas, where they have little natural protection from the problems of heat, drought and a plethora of new pests.

In other, more rare, cases a mutation might result in an abnormal protein that is still able to function but in a slightly different way from normal. While this is also most likely to prejudice the success of the organism, there is the converse possibility that it might actually present the organism with a more effective means of survival and reproductive success, either in the prevailing environmental conditions, or, more critically, when confronted with environmental changes that may be more hostile. For example, mutations are known that endow house-flies with resistance to the insecticide DDT, but, under the environmental conditions that prevailed before the use of DDT, these mutations slightly impaired the ability of the flies to grow and were generally disadvantageous. However, when DDT was introduced into the environment, the balance was tipped in favour of the mutant flies, which then became dominant in the population as a result of natural selection.

## Evolutionary change takes place over immense timescales

An important aspect of the evolutionary process that is sometimes difficult to grasp is its immense timescale. From the fossil record, it is possible to estimate that it has been 5 million years since the first apelike ancestors of man appeared on the planet and 34 million years since the first modern mammals, including apes, emerged. Although the first dinosaurs and early mammals inhabited the earth around 245 million years ago, the first primitive animals appeared as many as 560 million years ago. The oldest fossils of all, those of primitive microbes, date back as far as 3,500 million years. The earth is approximately 4,600 million years old and the universe itself is believed to have originated from the Big Bang of 15,000 million years ago.

It is extremely difficult to form any realistic idea of such vast stretches of time. From a personal view, our experiences extend back over tens of years, yet even for that limited period we are prone to forgetting precisely what the world was like when we were young. A hundred years ago, the earth was full of people all going about their daily business, yet, with only a very few exceptions, none of them is alive today. The brevity of human life limits the span of our direct personal recollection, yet we have illusions that our memories go further back than that. Human culture has given us a legacy of historical writings, as well as stories and myths passed down orally or in the form of pictures and carvings. With such aids we can, with some effort, project back around 4,000 years to get some idea of what the ancient civilizations of Egypt, the Middle East, Central America and China, and even some more primitive settlements, were like. However, our minds are not really built to deal easily with periods as long as even thousands of years, so that the immensity of time involved in the evolution of humans is really beyond our ready comprehension. To get around this conceptual difficulty, we often resort to comparisons such as equating the age of the earth with a single week of time. On this scale, the age of the universe since the Big Bang would be roughly two or three weeks, and the oldest animals would have been alive just over a day ago. Modern humans would have appeared only in the last ten seconds. It is only within this temporal context that we can reasonably address the question of whether the present changes in environmental conditions will influence the future evolution of humankind.

## Are fears for future generations exaggerated?

The environmental changes that seriously concern us at the moment have only been going on for an infinitesimally short time when compared with the vast scale of evolutionary time. It is only 150 years or so since the Industrial Revolution and just under 60 years since the end of World War II. There has been nothing like the time required for the mechanisms of natural selection to operate on human beings, even if the extent of mutation within our sperm and eggs were to have increased dramatically over the last hundred years or so. Worrying that man-made mutagens pose a serious evolutionary threat seems, on the available evidence, to be premature. A study of mutations inherited by the children of survivors of the atomic bombs dropped on the Japanese cities of Hiroshima and Nagasaki in 1945 revealed no significant increase over the levels detected in matched controls. In addition, there is as yet no really convincing evidence that tobacco smoking, a habit known to bathe the internal organs of smokers in a veritable soup of mutagens, actually induces mutations in sperm or eggs. Indeed, there is little data to suggest that any external agent increases the level of mutations in these particular cells. Such findings are quite surprising, but it has been argued that human sperm and egg cells are somehow relatively resistant to mutation. This may be because they have more powerful protection systems or highly efficient DNA repair systems, when compared with somatic cells. In this context, it will be recalled that the human body has the capacity to destroy cells with seriously defective DNA, by the processes of programmed cell death (see Chapter 10). This may well be applied in a particularly rigorous way to defective egg and sperm cells, thus preventing their participation in any fertilization processes. In any event, of the several million eggs made in ovaries and the four trillion sperm manufactured in the testes over a lifetime, only an infinitesimally small minority would ever be involved in the production of a baby. In addition, a considerable proportion of abnormal embryos and fetuses are spontaneously aborted. More than 50 per cent of embryos perish in the early stages of pregnancy. In summary, we have in place a number of screening processes to safeguard the genetic interests of future generations.

In general, any prognostications about mutations and human evolution in the light of present environmental changes are probably pointless at the moment. Rather than threatening our evolutionary future, a more likely outcome is that the present environmental changes will have much more immediate deleterious effects on the quality of our lives. As well as causing cancers, many air pollutants are also responsible for a range of respiratory problems. Solar radiation can cause severe sunburn and skin cancers, and many industrial chemicals are both toxic and carcinogenic. Nuclear radiation can kill but also induce radiation sickness; damage bone marrow, spleen, lymph nodes and blood cells; and also cause infertility.

A goodly proportion of the mutations we inherit from our parents appear to have arisen spontaneously, rather than through external environmental agents. These could have occurred as a result of DNA-copying errors at some stage, or possibly through attack by free radicals generated within cells. Some of these mutations manifest themselves as inherited diseases. Since the beginning of the last century, it has been known that various diseases are passed from parent to offspring. In general, when a disease is inherited, it is usually caused by an abnormality in a single protein arising from the inheritance of a gene carrying a mutation. For example, cystic fibrosis suffers have a defect in the gene that encodes a protein crucial for the transport of chloride ions in cells. Muscular dystrophy victims inherit a gene defect that results in the manufacture of a faulty muscle protein. Haemophiliacs inherit defects in the blood proteins that are essential for blood clotting. These are just a few examples of over a thousand inherited diseases currently known. This number will undoubtedly grow, as our clinical knowledge and ability to detect them increase. Whether the frequency of inherited diseases is rising in the face of increased levels of environmental mutagens must remain a matter of speculation for the present. There are simply insufficient data available to make any judgement. However, it is hard to see how any such inherited diseases could confer any competitive advantages. On the face of it, some seem highly disadvantageous in terms of natural selection: muscular dystrophy, cystic fibrosis and haemophilia, for example, as well as others that predispose victims to childhood cancers or heart disease. Nonetheless, there are some known exceptions. Victims of sickle-cell anaemia carry a mutation that affects the structure of their haemoglobin (a protein in red blood cells that is responsible for carrying oxygen from the lungs to tissues). As a result, the ability of suffers to survive in conditions of low oxygen (for example, at high altitudes) is impaired. Nevertheless they seem to have a considerable resistance to developing malaria, which may be a distinct advantage in certain environments. The sickle-cell gene has therefore persisted, rather than disappeared, due to natural selection.

History has proved that, over the relatively short span of our existence on earth, we are good survivors, but, like the dinosaurs, we could still succumb to environmental changes that are severely hostile and relatively rapid. Genes good for one environment can turn out to be less than ideal in another. Should our planet become seriously contaminated with pollutants, or the levels of solar radiation increase to unacceptable levels, it would become imperative to acquire genes that would confer increased resistance to chemical mutagens and harmful radiation. Because the processes of natural selection function far too slowly, a possible solution would be to resort to some type of gene technology in order to safeguard future generations of humankind. The next chapter considers some of these possibilities.

---

**Key points in this chapter**

- Darwin theorized that species were not specially created in their present form but that they evolved from ancestral species by natural selection.
- Organisms evolve to possess attributes that favour their survival and reproduction in the prevailing environmental conditions.
- Offspring can only inherit mutations induced in the DNA of sperm or eggs. In contrast, mutations in the DNA of somatic cells cannot be inherited.
- Inherited mutations can affect survival and reproductive success, and the slight differences between individuals in a population serve as the raw material for natural selection.
- Natural selection and evolutionary change take place over immense timescales.
- Taking account of the apparent resistance of human sperm and eggs to mutation by external agents and other safeguards that the human body has in place, fears regarding our long-term evolutionary fate in the face of present environmental threats are probably unwarranted at the present time.
- A more likely outcome is that the present environmental changes will have more immediate health effects, some of which may manifest themselves as cancers and other debilitating conditions.
- Ultimately these health effects may become so severe that gene technology may be considered as a possible solution.

---

# Genes to take the strain

The idea of a quick genetic fix that would allow us, like Superman with 'a leap and a bound', to short-circuit natural selection and survive severely hostile environmental conditions seems at first sight the stuff of science fiction, rather than reality. However, in view of the large amount of accumulated knowledge of genes and their manipulation that we have acquired in the last fifty years, the potential feasibility of such approaches merits some consideration.

Are there any genes available from any organisms, anywhere, that might allow us to take the strain of severe environmental change and emerge relatively unscathed? Since life first emerged on earth, all organisms have been exposed to environments that have, in the main, altered gradually, but also, from time to time, quite rapidly. Over millions of years, adaptation to environmental change has been possible through the twin processes of mutation and natural selection. On earth today there some very unwelcoming environments, but also living things adapted for successful life in these locations. Organisms called *extremophiles* are able to function in what seem to us extremely harsh environments. These particular organisms resemble bacteria, with which they have some genes in common, but they also have many unique genes. These are of great interest because they encode special proteins that allow the organisms to survive and function in extreme environments. For instance, the *thermophiles* inhabit hot springs at temperatures between 48 and 80 degrees Celsius. *Hyperthermophiles* thrive at even higher temperatures, between 80 and 150 degrees Celsius, again in hot springs, but also in undersea hydrothermal vents (black smokers). Others, like the *psychrophiles*, are adapted to the chilly temperatures (4 to 12 degrees Celsius) of the Antarctic sea-ice or ocean. Whereas *acidophiles* grow in the acidic conditions of some deep-sea hydrothermal vents, *alkaliphiles* inhabit alkaline soda lakes and carbonate-rich soils. Salt lakes or solar evaporation ponds provide a home for yet another group, the *halophiles*. At the moment, commercial organizations are keen to isolate some of the special proteins made by these unusual organisms in large quantities, for use in industrial processes. The aim is to capitalize on their ability not just to promote chemical reactions useful in commercial processes but also to do so at high or low temperatures, or in extremes of acidity or alkalinity. A very attractive feature regarding their likely use in this context is that they are environmentally clean. From the scientific point of view, a key question is, how can the proteins of the extremophiles manage to remain operational under conditions that would be lethal for most organisms? In the case of thermophiles, we know that, although many of their proteins are quite similar to those in normal heat-sensitive organisms, they often have more chemical bonds and other internal stabilizing forces, which means that they do not undergo debilitating changes at high temperatures.

Despite the obvious possibilities of commercial exploitation, it is doubtful as yet whether any of the genes for these special proteins of the extremophiles would be of direct value to man in any efforts to escape serious environmental adversity. There is, however, another group of genes that merit closer attention in this context. Collectively they are known as the *stress genes*, and they have evolved in a wide range of bacteria, animals and plants to provide a rapid response to environmental threats. The proteins produced from these genes play key roles that enable organisms to survive different types of environmental onslaught. These responses to stress are orchestrated at the gene level, and, characteristically, can be induced both rapidly and repeatedly. They are thus particularly useful to organisms living under rapidly changing environmental circumstances. Because a large number of these responses are seen in organisms ranging from bacteria to humans, they are likely to have arisen soon after primitive cells first appeared on earth.

## Stress genes

Stress genes were first recognized some forty years ago. At that time, an Italian geneticist, Ferrucio Ritossa, then working in Naples, noticed that when the environmental temperature of fruit fly larvae was raised from the normal 25 degrees to 32 degrees Celsius their chromosomes appeared to bulge, or puff out, at certain specific locations. Because of the special nature of the chromosomes of these particular insect larvae, this puffing indicated the switching on of specific genes in response to the stress of elevated temperature. This was the beginning of a trail that led to the analysis of many ubiquitous cellular responses, involving the activation of genes encoding proteins that allow organisms to tolerate conditions of environmental adversity. There is now intense research activity aimed at elucidating the mechanisms whereby specific environmental threats are sensed, and how the activation of relevant stress genes is triggered. While the ability of organisms to alter the spectrum of active genes has significance for the adjustment to short-term changes in environmental conditions, the possession of a diversity of genes that encode potentially protective stress proteins may have crucial evolutionary significance. Variants of such genes could be selectively advantageous when populations of organisms are confronted with more long-term environmental changes that may be both stressful and hostile. The appreciation and understanding of the diversity of genes in all types of living organism that encode protective proteins are thus an important aspect of biodiversity. A biodiverse range of stress genes, governing graded responses to a range of environmental threats, could be a major asset for our future. It would provide a valuable gene bank, possibly containing many unique variants of stress genes that would provide the technological basis for any future genetic enhancement we might envisage. It is paradoxical that, just at the time when biodiversity is under threat, our technological ability to appreciate the detailed organization of genes is increasing. Unfortunately, once a species is lost from the wild, the opportunity to understand, and possibly harness, its genes, including those that respond to stress, is also lost.

## A catalogue of genes for various contingencies

The following section takes a number of potential environmental threats, and examines the genes that might allow organisms to cope with them.

### Excessive global warming

At present, temperatures are continually changing within the environment, both during the day and from season to season. These fluctuations can have a very significant impact on general cellular functions, as well as on the complex machinery responsible for respiration and photosynthesis. The observations of Ritossa in 1962 suggested that increased temperatures caused the activation of specific genes. Later work showed that these genes encoded proteins that were subsequently christened the *heat shock proteins*. It is important to realize that the phenomenon is not peculiar to fruit flies; it can be initiated in all organisms from bacteria to humans, and is sometimes referred to as the heat shock response.

Human cells die if exposed to temperatures in excess of 43 degrees Celsius. However, if human cells are exposed to elevated temperature, but below 43 degrees, there is a rapid reprogramming of cellular activities to ensure survival during the period of heat stress, the aim being to protect essential cell components against heat damage and to permit a recovery from high-temperature stress, and a rapid resumption of normal activities. Another outcome is that such cells can now more readily tolerate exposure to high temperatures. This is the phenomenon of *thermotolerance*, which coincides with the activation of the genes for the production of heat shock proteins. Human cells that are naturally heat resistant have notably high levels of heat shock proteins, and transfer of active genes for heat shock proteins to isolated human cells, grown in the laboratory, can reduce the sensitivity of these cells to the adverse effects of high temperature stress.

Although the functions of many heat shock proteins are still the subject of intense investigation, it is nonetheless clear that an important role is to prevent the alterations to the crucial three-dimensional structure of cell proteins that can readily occur in heat-stressed cells. When an egg is boiled, its protein components begin to coagulate. In much the same way, exposure to elevated temperatures would normally cause cell proteins to change their shape and lose their ability to function properly. However, if heat shock proteins are available, they can rush to the rescue of these susceptible proteins, and minimize any possible heat damage. Heat shock proteins have a special construction that allows them to form a brief, but intimate, partnership with heat-damaged proteins within cells, and, in the process, restores them to their original functional state. This ability to maintain cell proteins in their correct three-dimensional state is at the heart of heat shock protein function. Even in unstressed cells there is always a small amount of heat shock proteins present, whose job it is to form partnerships with key cell proteins, not only to ensure their proper structure but also to act as chaperones, ferrying them to their correct cell locations or teaming them up with yet other cell proteins to create complex systems. Heat exposure simply activates the genes for heat shock proteins, so increasing the cellular concentrations of heat shock proteins available for additional duties that are likely to ensue if many cell proteins are damaged by heat.

In the case of human cells, increased heat shock protein production is seen following continuous exposures to temperatures between 40 and 42 degrees Celsius. These temperatures would represent a very severe fever indeed, with anything higher causing the cessation of all protein manufacture and cell death. In plants there is a threshold temperature above which heat shock protein manufacture is increased. Threshold temperatures vary with plant species rather than with environment. Heat shock protein induction occurs in maize at 30 degrees Celsius, whereas millet requires temperatures of 40 degrees and above.

How, then, are heat shock genes activated? A crucial aspect is that not all the nucleotide sequences in DNA actually encode proteins. Certain sequences lying outside the coding regions of genes form part of the control mechanism by which the activity of specific genes can be adjusted (see Figure 2.7). Thus, not only do nucleotide sequences in DNA determine the type and structure of the proteins made by cells, they also comprise part of the machinery that controls the level to which these proteins are produced in response to cell requirements. Temperature stress is just one of a number of environmental influences that lead to the activation of certain genes. However, a common feature of these situations is that control of the relevant genes is exercised through special stress-sensing proteins. Once a stress has been sensed, these proteins proceed to interact with the control sequences ahead of the relevant stress genes. It is these interactions that trigger the increased decoding of the adjacent genes with the eventual production of increased amounts of the appropriate protein (see Figure 2.7).

In the case of heat shock gene activation, a complex sensor acts in response not to heat per se, but rather to the presence of damaged, or aberrant, proteins within the stressed cells. This is why it is not just the stress of elevated temperature that causes the increase in heat shock gene activity. Any stressful agent that damages cell proteins will do the trick. The list includes alcohol, some toxic metals, oxygen deprivation and a number of drugs.

## Ice Age conditions

How might we cope with severe drops in temperature? With the exception of mammals, most organisms have little control over their body temperatures and are vulnerable to the hazard of crystallization of water into ice in their cells and tissues. Ice causes physical injury to cells due to the forces of shearing, puncture or expansion. Initially, a freezing front sweeps through the extracellular spaces of an organism without actually penetrating cells. This, in itself, can result in extensive damage due to the osmotic stress, and consequent loss of water it causes, with cells shrinking to a fraction of their original volume.

Many organisms that cannot avoid exposure to subzero temperatures, for example by selecting their habitats or hibernating in sheltered sites, instead employ strategies to lower the temperature at which their cellular fluids freeze. The most sophisticated of these is the switching on of either *antifreeze protein* production or the production of *protectants* like ethylene glycol (commonly used in automobile antifreeze mixtures).

Antifreeze proteins have been best studied in cold-water marine fishes and cold-tolerant insects. They have a particular ability to absorb themselves onto an ice crystal lattice. Although they do not prevent ice formation, they break up the crystal growth planes and interfere with crystal growth and so lower freezing points. In the case of fish, this lowering in body fluids can be up to 1 or 1.5 degrees Celsius. The lowest temperature that a fish can experience is limited by the fact that it lives in water. Insects, on the other hand, can encounter much lower temperatures. The antifreeze proteins from insects are therefore more powerful, and can lower freezing points by as much as 6 to 9 degrees Celsius. Where even more powerful protection is necessary, organisms such as insects often manufacture *colligative protectants* such as ethylene glycol, or glycerol. In winter, these can often account for as much as 20 per cent of their body weight. Insects manufacture glycerol from sugar reserves laid down in summer; by using these in combination with antifreeze proteins, they can maintain their body fluids in a liquid state down to temperatures approaching minus 40 degrees Celsius.

A type of cold shock response has been noted in plants. Mechanisms have evolved that allow acclimatization to cold temperatures. For example, if temperate plants, such as winter cereals, experience a period of exposure to low temperatures, this will allow them to withstand a subsequent freezing stress. The process is complex and includes membrane changes, as well as increases in concentrations of compounds that have a role similar to that of glycerol in insects, together with the appearance of proteins, some of which have antifreeze properties. Many of these changes are under the control of *low-temperature responsive genes*. The outer membrane of plant cells is an important site of injury during freezing, but prior exposure of plants to low temperatures causes a subtle change in the fat composition of their membranes. This is brought about by stress genes that direct the inclusion of more unsaturated fatty acids into plant membranes, which makes them more tolerant of chilling temperatures.

## Conditions of severe drought

A number of genes are activated specifically by low-temperature treatment of plants. Significantly, many of these genes are also activated in conditions of drought. Since, during freezing, ice crystals form outside cells, freezing and droughting can both be viewed as dehydration stresses. Environmental conditions of high salinity or drought pose considerable threats to a variety of organisms. The productivity of many commercially grown agronomic and horticultural crops is usually adversely affected by high soil salinity and drought, and salt accumulation in soils caused by irrigation may ultimately inhibit the sustainability of agriculture. Under such conditions, cells of bacteria and plants are threatened with dehydration and respond by varying the chemical composition of their cells. They have sensors that detect changes in hydrostatic pressure. In turn, these regulate the switching on of genes that promote the manufacture of special chemicals that they can accumulate to very high concentrations, but that do not interfere with their general metabolism. Examples of such compounds that protect from dehydration are sugars (for example, trehalose), polyols (for example, glycerol), amino acids (for example, proline) and derivatives of amino acids (for example, glycine, betaine).

## Toxic metal pollution

A number of metals are nutritionally important and some, like zinc, can act to facilitate the action of a considerable number of important cell proteins, and are not normally toxic, even at extremely high concentrations. Indeed, zinc is found naturally in all growing organisms. Others, like copper, although also nutritionally important at low concentrations, are a problem at high concentrations. In contrast, metals such as cadmium and mercury are highly toxic and without nutritional value.

In biological systems, nutritionally important metals usually act to ensure a particular protein can adopt the correct shape necessary for it to function. They may also directly facilitate that function. The metals, or more correctly their ions, often resemble one another chemically, which can cause some significant problems in biological systems. Ions derived from cadmium and lead can compete with essential ions such as those from calcium or magnesium, and so block the function of several important cell proteins. Copper ions can substitute for important zinc ions and cause problems with the copying of DNA, and the reading of the genetic code.

The toxicity of mercury lies in the ability of ions derived from it to combine irreversibly with certain parts of protein molecules and block their proper function. Perhaps the most notorious case of mercury contamination occurred in Japan in the fishing village of Minamata, where a chemical factory producing acetaldehyde was built in the 1930s.

The industrial process unfortunately involved the use of mercury, and the mercury-laden waste was simply dumped into the nearby Minamata Bay. Bacteria converted the mercury to a compound called methyl mercury, which worked its way up the food chain in ever-increasing concentrations. By the 1940s, there were many unexplained deaths of fish in the local waters. In the 1950s the factory stepped up its production, together with the dumping of mercury. Not long after, many of the local cats appeared to go mad. They danced as if they were drunk, and then vomited and died. It was referred to as the 'cat dancing disease', but there was to be a more sinister turn. By 1956 children in the area began to suffer brain damage, a symptom of which was to become know as 'Minamata disease'. The problem was diagnosed as arising from eating mercury-contaminated fish. Nonetheless, despite attacks on the factory in 1959 by local fishermen, whose fish were, not surprisingly, impossible to sell, the factory continued to dump mercury in the bay for a further ten years. Thousands developed symptoms and at least a hundred victims died. Lawsuits were mounted and, by 1973, around $100 million was paid out to victims and their families. For many years, no one from elsewhere in Japan would marry anyone from Minamata. They were simply scared that such action would lead to deformed offspring. By 1984 the Japanese government was persuaded to decontaminate the floor of Minamata Bay by dredging, at the cost of around $400 million. Only in 1994 were they able to declare the area free of mercury and remove the netting set up in the 1970s to keep out unsuspecting fish. Thus ended probably the worst contamination of the sea in human history.

Like mercury, cadmium has no known beneficial effect on human health. It enters the environment from the burning of coal or household waste, as well as from cigarette smoke, metal mining and refining processes. It is also widely used in the production of batteries, metal coatings and plastics. If air with high levels of cadmium is inhaled, severe lung damage, and even lung cancer, can ensue, with the additional problem that, over many years, there can be a build-up of cadmium in the kidneys, leading to kidney disease. Recent studies with isolated human cells in the laboratory show that cadmium compounds can damage DNA by causing strand breaks, as well as by directly binding to DNA, and bring about cross-links between DNA strands.

These different types of damage can cause mutations and chromosomal abnormalities. Moreover, chromium compounds can also block the systems that are available within cells to repair any damaged DNA, and there is evidence to indicate that cadmium and cadmium compounds can cause cancer in humans.

Despite the toxicity problems associated with certain metals, bacteria, animals and plants all have systems that can sense toxic levels of metal ions and activate special genes that encode proteins that have a protective role. However, when it comes to coping with metals in the environment, bacteria are in the front line. The ease with which they can tolerate high concentrations of potentially toxic metals is truly impressive. Bacteria harbour genes that confer resistance to a variety of toxic elements including antimony, arsenic, boron, cadmium, chromium, copper, mercury, lead, nickel, silver, tellurium and zinc. Resistance of bacteria to mercury has been particularly well studied, and it turns out that toxic forms of mercury can be rendered less toxic through the activity of a number of bacterial proteins acting in concert. These proteins arise from a set of bacterial genes that can be activated by a sensor and respond to sub-lethal concentrations of mercury compounds. In the same way, other bacterial genes can be activated by sub-lethal levels of copper or cadmium, with the resultant production of appropriate copper or cadmium detoxification proteins.

In humans, the genes for *metallothioneins* are probably the best understood metal-activated genes. Although metallothioneins are very small proteins, they have an unusually high propensity to mop up certain metal ions. Their role in protecting us from the toxic effects of metals correlates with the ability of a number of metals such as lead, zinc, copper and cadmium to activate the decoding of their genes. For example, cadmium, which enters the body mainly by inhalation and ingestion, is a good inducer of metallothionein genes. The metallothioneins produced can subsequently bind to the offending cadmium, primarily in the liver and kidney, and it is in this harmless bound form that most of the cadmium intake is retained by the kidneys and liver. Whilst this storage can be for as long as twenty years or more, too great a cadmium intake can overload the available capacity and thus become a serious health hazard.

## Chemical pollution

Many synthetic and naturally occurring chemicals in the environment are stressful because they can cause severely adverse biological effects in the cells of animals and plants. Some protection from certain potentially toxic chemicals is nonetheless possible because of the ability of some organisms to switch on genes that encode detoxification proteins. These detoxification proteins can often directly reduce the toxicity of such harmful compounds, or increase their solubility in water as a first step towards their elimination from the afflicted organism (see also Chapters 5 and 9).

Although chemicals such as polycyclic aromatic hydrocarbons and halogenated aromatic hydrocarbons are generally bad news, they can nonetheless switch up the activity of genes encoding certain detoxifying proteins. If they gain access to cells, they are met by a special receptor protein. This encounter then signals up another protein, which, after joining them, facilitates their translocation to the appropriate control sequences in the DNA lying ahead of genes for a number of detoxifying proteins, including certain cytochrome P450s and glutathione adding proteins (see also Chapters 5 and 9). This causes the increased activation of these genes to augment the level of detoxification proteins available to meet new threats. As previously discussed, there is quite a large range of different cytochrome P450 types, so it is perhaps not too surprising that the actual category of cytochrome P450 gene activated varies with different toxic chemicals.

The possibility of causing the induction of detoxifying proteins with various drugs has triggered a growing interest in the possibilities of developing *chemointervention* strategies for human populations routinely exposed to cancer-causing agents. Aflatoxin B1 (see Chapter 6) is a potent dietary toxin that has been linked to liver cancers and to which humans are commonly exposed in several parts of the world. Aflatoxin B1 is initially acted upon in the liver by a member of the cytochrome P450 family. Rather than converting it to a harmless form, the cytochrome P450 transforms it to a highly reactive form that attacks guanine (G) nucleotides in DNA. Laboratory experiments, however, suggest a way out of this problem. Genes that encode a protein with the ability to couple glutathione (see Chapter 5 and 9) to the reactive form of aflatoxin B1, and so render it harmless, can be activated by the drug Oltipraz. Subsequent experiments have shown that treatment of rats with Oltipraz can protect these animals from the carcinogenic effects of aflatoxin B1. Based on these animal studies, drugs like Oltipraz are now being considered for human use as a means of similarly protecting against aflatoxin B1-induced liver cancers. Chemoprevention is also available at the dietary level. For example allyl sulphide and diallyl sulphide, present in garlic and onions, inhibit cytochrome P450 but activate the glutathione-coupling detoxification systems.

## Depletion of atmospheric oxygen

Perhaps the most extreme environmental stress for the majority of species is oxygen deprivation. In mammals, this can be a hazard for vital tissues that suffer either a partial or total deficiency in situations where blood supplies are impaired. For plants that are not appropriately adapted, flooded or waterlogged conditions, which carry with them the risk of severe oxygen deficiency, are also potentially detrimental. Deprivation of oxygen in animals and plants rapidly reduces their supply of energy-providing chemicals, and, although a period of oxygen deprivation can be survived, it can cause tissue death if prolonged.

Most plant species able to grow in flooded or waterlogged soils can survive the hazards of oxygen deprivation by highly developed aeration systems. Nonetheless, there are examples in less well-adapted plants of tissues such as seeds, root tips, regions of tree trunks, rhizomes and stolons, where the demand for oxygen often outstrips supply. In the roots of some crops under such conditions it has been possible to detect the activation of genes encoding a select group of stress proteins called the *anaerobic proteins*. Of the twenty or so such proteins, most appear to be proteins that promote the acquisition of energy from sugars under conditions that lack oxygen. Energy production under the stress of oxygen deficiency is thus a priority, and there is evidence for a sensor that detects such a contingency in plant tissues and switches on a set of appropriate genes.

In the cells of mammals a notable feature of oxygen deprivation is the activation of the gene for the growth regulating protein, p53.

Although the mechanism involved is not fully understood, there appears to be a sensor protein that stabilizes p53 and, in turn, facilitates the activation of several genes sometimes referred to as the *oxygen regulated protein genes*. The precise roles that proteins from such genes might have in oxygen-deprived cells are, however, still the subject of ongoing investigations, although at least two appear to function in the arrest of normal cell division. Such a response may be advantageous in terms of energy conservation in conditions of limited oxygen.

## Excessive solar radiation

Damage from solar radiation is likely to become ecologically significant as a consequence of reductions to the stratospheric ozone layer. However, in terms of possible stress genes, the responses in human cells to excessive ultraviolet radiation are still very much under investigation and appear to be complex. As already discussed in Chapter 8, a consequence of the inevitable DNA damage is the activation of the gene encoding the p53 protein. This protein has a key role in orchestrating the complex cell responses to DNA damage. However, preliminary research shows that a number of other genes are also activated in human cells in response to intense ultraviolet radiation. Notable among these is one that encodes a protein called *haem oxygenase*. This protein appears to facilitate the conversion of certain types of molecule, produced from the breakdown of blood cells pigments, into forms that can act as antioxidants. Because ultraviolet radiation of skin, besides damaging DNA, also causes the release of free radicals, the creation of extra antioxidant protection by this route could be significant. Another response to solar radiation is the production of *melanin*, which is the cause of skin tanning. This black polymer is manufactured in human skin from an amino acid called tyrosine after exposure to strong sunlight and provides some UVB protection. A skin cell protein, tyrosinase, promotes the first step in the process, but some of the subsequent polymerization reactions may be facilitated by free radicals released when skin is exposed to ultraviolet light.

While solar radiation in the visible range of the spectrum is an absolute requirement for plant life, there is a wide diversity in plant resistance to the damaging effects of ultraviolet radiation. Although visible signs of ultraviolet damage in the field are rare, experiments have been carried out under conditions intended to mimic the levels of ultraviolet radiation that might be encountered following severe stratospheric ozone depletion. Plants respond to such conditions with the activation of genes for the manufacture of protective flavonoids in the outer layers of leaves with a resultant bronzing or reddening.

---

**Key points in this chapter**

- Stress-resistant proteins exist in extremophiles. These organisms thrive at extremes of temperatures, at extremes of acidity or alkalinity, or in extremely salty conditions. In the future, their stress-resistant proteins may be used in industrial processes, as they are environmentally clean.

- All living organisms contain a variety of stress genes whose activation follows exposure to a range of environmental threats. This leads to the production of special cell stress proteins that play important roles in helping organisms resist, or tolerate, particular environmental adversities.

- The products of these stress genes include heat shock proteins (which confer thermal resistance and repair damaged cell proteins), antifreeze proteins, and regulators of osmotic pressure, metallothioneins and proteins to detoxify metals, chemical detoxifying proteins, ultraviolet protectors, and so on.

---

# 14

# Gene attacks by humans

*Genetic engineering is new threat to sport* was a recent headline in a local newspaper. The article's author was genuinely concerned at the spectre of a nightmare team of genetically engineered giant basketball players, or squad of sprinters who could make present world record holders look puny and pedestrian. He was clearly distressed at the sprint pace of scientific progress, his views probably stemming from much press speculation that designer babies may soon be a real possibility. His concern originates from the steady progress from the discoveries, beginning in the 1970s, that genes could not only be isolated but also be moved to create combinations that had never been seen before in nature. Other milestones along that route have been the development of *in vitro* fertilization techniques some twenty-five years ago, and the birth in 1996 of Dolly the clone, perhaps the most famous lamb in the world. This has all been a part of an attack on genes in which mankind could be viewed as the aggressor. Human desires for perfect babies are understandable and market forces may well push research in that direction, but the possibility still exists that these advances could provide us with possibilities other than great height for prowess in basketball, or stature and musculature appropriate for sprinting. As mentioned in the previous chapter, a more long-sighted view might be that the technology could be used to devise new genetic combinations that would open up the possibility of short-circuiting natural selection in order to survive possible future catastrophic changes in the environment.

## The great gene robbery

For some considerable time, and even before the advent of genetic engineering, humans have been in the business of gene robbery. The wheat we use for pasta and bread is an example. Its ancestral forms still grow in the fertile crescent of the Middle East. Rice, now grown all over the warmer world, originated in Southeast Asia, and corn, a principal food plant of the Western world, came from Central America. All of these staple crops are in fact hybrid varieties, the products of intense crossing and selection by plant breeders over thousands of years. To keep these hybrids healthy and productive, we have to return regularly to their native countries to extract genes from their wild relatives by plant breeding. In essence, we have become gene robbers 'stealing' from the world's precious resource of genetic diversity.

Modern potato varieties bear little resemblance to their Peruvian ancestors. In Peru and Ecuador there are over 150 different species of potato occurring naturally. From these the Incas, Aztecs and Quechuas, over the last thousand years, selected and bred new seed stock, managing to cultivate at last three thousand different varieties. By planting a crop comprising a dozen or more of these varieties at a time, they found that, should diseases strike, only part of the crop would succumb. The danger of relying on a single variety is that if one plant falls victim, for example, to a fungal disease, then the remainder of the crop will very shortly be afflicted. A classic example of just such a situation is writ large in the pages of Irish history. In 1846, during the Irish potato famine, around a million people died of starvation. A number of political, commercial and scientific factors were contributory. However, a notable feature was a lack of species diversity in the potato crop of the time. This meant that no potato plants in the Irish fields were resistant to the blight caused by the fungus *Phytophthora infestans*. This resulted in a growth of white mould on the leaves and eventually turned the potatoes into a white, toxic mush. Despite this, the commercial pressures of present times still dictate genetic uniformity. Even in the UK, 50 per cent of the potatoes produced are from just five varieties. However, to keep even the Peruvian varieties healthy, it is necessary to maintain the genetic resource of their ancestors in the wild. The genetic diversity of potatoes is so precious that a gene bank in the shape of the International Potato Centre has been established outside Lima, in Peru. Not only is valuable genetic stock stored there but also work continues on the development of further potato varieties, by crossing wild and cultivated varieties. Higher up in the Andes, thousands of different varieties are planted out every year so as to keep up a living bank of genes. Today, potato breeders from the richer countries of the world can visit these gene banks, and, for a fee, dip into what is a Third World genetic resource, returning home with novel varieties from which they can breed potatoes that more closely match their particular climatic and specialized commercial requirements. Financial support for such gene banks comes mainly from Western countries, and their operation requires the rigorous control of security, as well as of trading conditions. However, the gene banks could easily run dry. The vital wild varieties are always under threat from land destruction by developers, road builders and even farmers themselves. Moreover, the gene banks themselves are in danger, not just from simple catastrophes such as power cuts, which could affect vital refrigeration machinery, but also from the more insidious issues of local political and civil strife. This subtle form of gene robbery is not just confined to potatoes; similar issues relate to wheat, maize, rice and beans. The gene banks of the Third World operate just to keep Western countries supplied, or even oversupplied, with food.

The genetic improvement of plants by these methods involves a process where human interference essentially guides the evolution of varieties. It is artificial selection rather than natural selection. Farmers or breeders may artificially select for characteristics that, although potentially disadvantageous in nature, may be deemed advantageous to man. As a result, the genetic make-up of a cultivated crop plant may become gradually more and more removed from that of its wild ancestors. A key point is that artificial selection advances at a rate faster than natural selection because it is significantly directed.

## Genetic engineering: progress or evolutionary vandalism?

The breeding of crops and domestic animals by the traditional methods of artificial selection will undoubtedly continue in years to come, producing many improvements from the human perspective. In the end, however, it is constrained by the limitations of sexual compatibility, which prevents the cross-breeding of separate species. However, since the advent of genetic engineering in 1973 this barrier has been lifted. This technique, developed by Stanley Cohen and Herbert Boyer, along with others, allows the breeder to snip out genes from one species and place them in the DNA of another, possibly quite unrelated, species. The first genetic engineering experiments succeeded in putting working foreign genes into the bacterium *E. coli*, which normally lives in the human gut. Because of these foreign genes now inside them, the bacteria took on different characteristics. The transplanted genes gave *E. coli* resistance to certain antibiotics. However, the organisms, with their new properties, were not dangerous, and were readily wiped out by other antibiotics. The experiment was completely safe, and such biotechnological achievements led to the growth of a new set of industries, particularly in the USA, the UK and Japan.

Many scientists nonetheless became concerned that moving genes from one bacterium to another could cause outbreaks of new infectious diseases, or even environmental disasters. Concerned scientists urged a temporary halt in genetic experimentation until the scientific community could debate the hazards, and produce some sort of guidelines to ensure safe working practices and prevent accidents. A now famous conference was held in Asilomar, California, in 1975 specifically to debate these issues. This brought a sense of reason to a situation that had initially seemed fraught with potential dangers. After the Asilomar conference, scientists proceeded with considerable caution and a set of guidelines was established for carrying out genetic engineering experiments with a number of safety review boards and procedures being put in place.

Genetic engineering allows genes to cross the species barrier, and thereby extends the potential for crop and livestock improvement by creating new genetic material for breeders to work with. One view is that it is simply an extension of normal breeding methods, but there are others who see it as a special situation requiring rigorous control. Although the guidelines facilitated safe progress, a number of issues still worry the public at large. In the context of food and agriculture, it continues to be a battle for hearts and minds, despite the sincere belief of many big multinational companies that the application of genetic engineering would be greeted with enthusiasm in the market-place. They were genuinely convinced that there would be many beneficial effects for crop production and the environment. The first genetically engineered products eaten by humans were cheese and tomatoes. Genetically engineered bacteria were initially used to produce an alternative means of making cheese, which resulted in a purely vegetarian product. Then, in 1995, tomatoes with their 'softening gene' switched off, so that they could ripen on the vine to reach their full flavour and colour without rotting, were introduced into the market place in the form of tomato paste. Subsequently, the greatest efforts have been put into engineering crops that can tolerate herbicides or insect pests. These crops include soya, oilseed rape, maize, sugar beet and cotton. It was believed that success in these areas would see a great reduction in the use of herbicides and insecticides, which would have considerable benefits for the environment. Moreover, there was a genuine, almost evangelistic, view that the advances in genetic engineering would ultimately help in feeding the developing world. In the future, crops could well be engineered to resist climatic conditions that lead to famine, or to require less input of fertilizers. Certainly, the prospects for feeding the world, which undoubtedly does face a food production challenge using other current technologies, do not inspire confidence. In Africa, for example, per capita food production has already fallen by 20 per cent since the mid-1960s. But feeding the world is not a simple problem with a simple solution, even though enough food is produced worldwide to feed everyone adequately. Poverty is an important factor. Poor countries would simply not be able to afford the expensive modern technologies offered that would theoretically improve their yields. It has been argued that a better alternative would be to provide relatively modest financial resources, simply to make the older technologies more readily available and thus improve farms and livelihoods by more conventional means. Although genetically engineered crops could make a contribution to food quantity and quality, both in industrialized and developing countries, big questions remain to be addressed.

Whilst the commercial organizations involved were familiar with some of these arguments, it came as a severe shock to them to learn that a significantly large proportion of the public actually felt that genetically engineered food products were in some way contaminated. Despite strict regulation and a clean safety record, the development of genetically engineered crops and other organisms has met with tremendous public hostility. Some public apprehensions are not without foundation; these have already been outlined in Chapter 6. It has to be conceded, even by the most ardent enthusiasts, that the insertion of foreign genes into an organism could well have long-term, unpredictable biological effects. One potential risk is that the present technology is unable to transplant foreign genes to precise locations in the recipient's chromosomes. An incoming gene is essentially 'parachuted in', and its final landing spot might easily be in the middle of, or close to, genes that are important for the normal functioning of that organism. The untargeted gene could then be the cause of minor, or even quite major, perturbations to the existing delicate genetic programming of the recipient. Another concern is that unusual proteins, or more than the normal amounts of natural plant toxins, could be produced. These might prove toxic for the consumer, or cause allergic reactions. However, it is possible by rigorous experimentation and testing to evaluate many of the issues that have arisen in the public debates, which at times have become very heated. The results of such tests will go part of the way in determining the future for this emerging technology.

A real threat to any future progress, however, is the very genuine public concern over the moral acceptability of genetic engineering. In this case it is not our own genes that are under siege. Instead we have now laid siege to millions of years of genetic evolutionary history. Deep down, many see the technology as an unwarranted attack by humans on the genes of other species. We could be viewed as gene vandals, able to steal genes from their rightful owners and, in moving them to new locations, deliberately create new genetic combinations that have never been seen in nature before. Have we the right to counteract, irreversibly, the perceived evolutionary wisdom of millions of years? Ideological battle lines have been drawn up between those who thrive on the very idea of progress and those who reject it, sometimes out of hand. The debate will undoubtedly continue. There is no going back: the gene genie is well and truly out of the bottle. We cannot 'undiscover' genetic engineering, but it may well be a Faustian bargain for humankind. Already, the less acceptable face of genetic engineering is apparent, as the threat of genetically engineered strains of viruses and bacteria used as weapons for bioterrorism has now become a reality. As the physicists found to their cost in relation to the problems of nuclear fission, biologists have now to accept that they can no longer be considered altogether trustworthy, and worldwide control is impossible. Rather than bland assurances on the wonders of inevitable progress and the search for ultimate truths, they have to accept responsibility firmly and defend their actions to the public.

## Gene medicine

Where do we go now? We cannot step back in time and 'undiscover' our ability to snip out genes and move them between species. Public opinion may turn against future progress. Whilst this could well be the case for genetically engineered food products, paradoxically there is still a hint of public approval for the manufacture of medicines, such as insulin and blood-clot-destroying proteins, using genetic engineering. Moreover, there is considerable public interest in the possibility of using gene therapy to correct the problems of inherited human disease. Even when genetic counselling and prenatal diagnosis are fully available to families that are known to have an inherited disorder, more often than not they have a deep-seated hope that, by replacing their defective gene with the normal one, albeit 'cannibalized' from another human being, it might be possible to cure members of the family that are already afflicted. Even with the early optimism of scientists for this possibility, considerable obstacles to success were readily admitted. Safe means of introducing a normal gene into the appropriate cells would have to be devised, as well as the means of ensuring that the particular gene was active within these cells. The first clinical trials of gene therapy for patients with a mutation in the gene that encodes a protein called *adenosine deaminase* were begun in 1990. The victims, mainly children, suffer a condition known as *severe combined immunodeficiency*. They are unable to mount the normal immune responses to infections, and have to lead a highly restricted life, usually in a specially constructed sterile environment, to be safe from dangerous infectious agents, hence the alternative description of the condition as 'baby in the bubble' syndrome. Without very intensive care, they usually die before two years of age. In the trials, white blood cells were first removed from the children, and then infected with a virus that was genetically engineered to carry the normal gene for adenosine deaminase. The treated cells were then returned to the patients. The children subsequently received gene-corrected cells every one to two months for up to a year, and did show signs of clinical improvement, although there was no permanent cure. Some ten years later, a more sophisticated approach was developed in which a special class of pre-cursor white blood cells, called stem cells, is first isolated from the bone marrow of victims. These cells can then be genetically engineered to correct the gene defect and the returned to the patient, where they give rise to a continuous supply of mature white blood cells capable of combating infectious agents. Although this approach has been much more successful in terms of increasing the victim's quality of life, there have been serious setbacks. When one of the patients in the US developed chickenpox, his immune system, as expected, attempted to ward off infection by increasing his white blood cell count. However, some of these cells continued to divide out of control, and he is now being tested for leukaemia. A second child in a French programme has also developed leukaemia-like symptoms. The upshot has been the cessation of gene therapy trials both in the US and in the UK.

Another target for gene therapy was the defective gene in victims of *cystic fibrosis*. The symptoms are due to a deficiency in their ability to deal with chloride ions within the tissues of the lung. This arises from mutations in a gene that encodes a protein, CFTR. Adenoviruses, which can cause a type of common cold, can infect the cells lining the air passages of our lungs very efficiently. This virus was genetically engineered to include the normal human CFTR gene, and so provide a means of introducing that gene specifically into the cells of the air passage cells of the cystic fibrosis patients. Unfortunately, with most of the varieties of adenovirus used, although the normal CFTR gene could be introduced into the patients' lung cells, it only seemed to remain active there for a limited period (two to three weeks). This puts severe limitations on the usefulness of this particular gene therapy.

Other viruses have been explored in the quest for better ways to insert normal genes into appropriate defective target cells. One group, the retroviruses, have the advantage that, unlike the adenoviruses, they can actually insert the normal gene directly into the DNA of the target cells. This means that all the progeny cells arising from the initial infected cell would also carry the inserted gene. The disadvantage, however, is that retroviruses can only insert the new gene randomly. Although the inserted genes usually work, the random insertion may lead to the disruption of other genes and/or their operation within the recipient cells. At the moment, this presents unacceptable risks. Another problem with retroviruses is that it is technically difficult to accumulate sufficient quantities in the laboratory to infect a significant number of cells in the tissues of a human patient. These problems severely limit their potential usefulness. The development of more efficient and precise ways of delivering genes to the cells of interest and controlling their activity remains a major challenge.

Besides the many technical problems, there are also various ethical and societal issues that need to be explained to, and discussed with, the public at large. For instance, it is important to distinguish between gene therapies that involve somatic cells as opposed to sex cells. Gene therapy involving somatic cells could be used to treat a patient already afflicted. The result, if all went well, would be a genetic change that is confined to the patient alone. In many ways it is analogous to the treatment of a genetic disorder with an organ or tissue transplant. Gene therapy involving eggs, however, is quite a different story. It is controversial, because any gene modification would be passed on to the children of the treated patient. Some groups see this as unethical, because we do not have such a right to impose such an alteration on our descendants, however good our intentions. On the other hand, it is clear that some parents may well be very keen to participate in a process that would forever banish the deleterious mutation from their family. The key question is, does the potential elimination of human misery outweigh the risks involved in gene therapy?

To a certain extent, addressing these issues is somewhat premature. So far gene therapy has proved to be one of medicine's greatest disappointments. No cures for inherited disease have yet emerged. In some cases it has even made patients worse. More worryingly still, one victim recently died following the injection of an adenovirus carrying a gene to treat a liver disorder. This death could have resulted from an inflammatory response to the virus preparation, which may have spread away from the intended target liver cells. Despite these set-backs, gene therapy has not been abandoned. Some medical research-ers still remain surprisingly optimistic, but much remains to be learned.

## A new way of making babies

In 1996 a clone was born. The creation of Dolly the lamb, stemming from the work of Ian Wilmut in the Roslin Institute, near Edinburgh, was a momentous event in the evolution of life on earth. This was a totally different way of making babies. The normal routes of fertiliza-tion, which have been evolved over millions of years of evolutionary history, could apparently be short-circuited. The technique of cloning was novel because it could create a baby from a single cell rather than requiring the participation of a father's sperm cell and a mother's egg cell in the complex processes of fertilization. The result, however, was simply a genetic copy and, despite the intense media furore surround-ing Dolly, nothing genetically new was created.

Not surprisingly, the event rapidly sparked off frenzied speculation about the possibilities of cloning humans. Scenarios of duplicate hu-mans and raising the dead that would not look out of place in science fiction were invoked. On the positive side, it was claimed that the technique may well have real benefits, particularly for infertile couples. Religious groups quickly rushed to the barricades, saying that cloning, which would put humanity in the position of being its own creator, was abhorrent. Although the World Health Organization was also opposed to human cloning, other groups, which included gay men and women, were not so adversely disposed to the exciting possibilities of cloning themselves. Nonetheless, US President Clinton was quick to request that the National Bioethics Advisory Commission undertake a thorough review of the legal and ethical issues involved. There were worries that individuals might be cloned without their consent, or that people would seek to clone those with great intellectual powers, beauty, athletic prowess or even outstanding basketball skills. There was concern that our evolutionary future was suddenly 'up for grabs'. Rather than creating genetic diversity, which is the feedstock for the processes of natural selection, cloning would tend to create genetic uniformity. This could have distinct evolutionary disadvantages. For instance, such populations could be uniformly susceptible to the ravages of novel diseases and less able to withstand various environmental challenges.

Setting aside these arguments, it is nonetheless clear that the idea of cloning humans has kindled a great deal of enthusiasm as well as hostility. Are we on the threshold of something that is both dangerous and wrong? The techniques used intervene in one of the most intimate processes of life. But for infertile couples it may appear to be a medical miracle. In their minds, unwilling to countenance any disadvantages, it would be the chance to have children of their own. However, at this time, in the UK and in thirty-nine other countries, human cloning is banned. This, of course, does not rule out the possibility that human cloning will be attempted in countries lacking such legislation. Although prevention of human cloning will not be easy, there may be a number of significant technical and biological barriers to success, with the result that public enthusiasm may wane in the long run.

Although there has perhaps been a tendency to play them down, there certainly are barriers to human cloning. For over thirty years scientists in various countries have tried to clone animals from adult cells but without success. By the 1980s, many of those involved felt that it was simply impossible. Nature seemed to have imposed its own roadblock on further progress. Then, quite suddenly, it seems that whatever obstacles prevented any advancement over these years magically vanished due to the use of slightly different techniques. The procedure used by Ian Wilmut and his colleagues involves first taking an egg from the womb and removing its nucleus, which contains its entire DNA. This leaves a hollow egg, devoid of any genetic material. A cell from the adult to be cloned is then isolated. In the case of a human this could be from the cheek pouch swab or from a small tissue biopsy. The nucleus, containing the DNA from this adult cell, is removed and transplanted into the empty egg. The egg, with this implanted genetic material from the adult to be cloned, is then stimulated to grow using mild electric shock treatment, as well as stimulatory chemicals. The general aim of these treatments, which are central to Wilmut's approach, is to switch the adult cell back to becoming the first cell of life. From this initial state, the egg, after a few days, grows to the embryo stage on a dish supplied with special growth substances. If this is successful, the embryo is then transplanted into the womb of the surrogate mother, where, if all goes well, it may ultimately become an infant animal. Thus far, only animals have been cloned: sheep, goats, cattle and mice, and even in expert hands the technique is far from efficient. Success is difficult to repeat. Out of a hundred sheep eggs implanted with adult genes, only two to three clones are usually achieved. Most fail to give rise to embryos, or simply fail to develop when implanted in the womb. Of really serious concern were observations that a considerable number of cloned lambs showed signs of abnormalities. Dolly herself developed acute arthritis as well as signs of premature ageing and was put down in 2003. Around the world many animal clones were reported to be dying of bizarre and inexplicable conditions. Many had deformities never before encountered in the veterinary world. These involved problems with breathing, and other pulmonary problems, abnormalities of musculature, as well as cardiac and immunological irregularities. Before any attempts to clone humans proceed, these warning signs cannot be ignored and need to be further investigated. The implications for human cloning are ominous; human clones, should they be produced, are very likely to suffer diseases as yet unknown to human medicine. In any event, although human embryo research is permitted in the UK, it is only allowed up until the fourteen-day stage, which would preclude attempts to evaluate the difficulties as far as humans are concerned, at least in the UK.

Notwithstanding these very loud alarm signals, researchers in some parts of the world are vying to create the first cloned human. Already an Italian fertility specialist has claimed on a television show that three women are pregnant with cloned babies. More bizarre was the announcement of a cloned baby by the leaders of a religious cult that believes human life was created by extraterrestrials. At the time of writing, it has been impossible to evaluate any of these claims and most responsible scientists have greeted them with scepticism and condemnation. Indeed, the United Nations set up a panel in 2001 aimed at drafting an international treaty to ban the cloning of human beings for the present. Although drafting of such a treaty could take some time, these startling claims may well help to accelerate the legislative processes involved. If there is to be any progress at all in the area of human cloning, it should be achieved cautiously with internationally agreed guidelines and rigorous regulation.

The natural process of human fertilization has been honed to its present state of efficiency over many years of evolutionary time. It may be grossly arrogant of us to expect crude means of short-circuiting its safeguards, such as cloning, to work without problems. A critical stage in the process appears to lie in the need to reset, or reprogramme, in some subtle way, the implanted adult DNA to make it behave as if it were the DNA of a normally fertilized egg and about to commence the processes of development to the embryo stage and beyond. We have still to learn how this actually takes place, and to control it properly, rather than leaving matters to chance using the somewhat hit-or-miss techniques of electric shock and chemical treatment. There are indications that a key to this mystery lies in subtle chemical changes that are superimposed upon the structure of DNA as cells reach the adult stage. Some of the nucleotide units in the DNA sequence that control the activity of genes are modified by the addition of small chemical entities called methyl groups. These appear to add an extra layer of regulation to the business of switching genes off and on. To return to the egg stage from the adult condition, these natural modifications to DNA have to be undone, or reset. This problem may well explain the lack of cloning success in the thirty years that preceded the appearance of Dolly.

Cloning humans may be even more challenging than first supposed. Although there have been reports of cloned human embryos, these embryos have only developed as far as the six-cell stage. This may be due to problems similar to those experienced by groups attempting to clone monkeys, which, like us, are primates. Whilst the monkey embryos looked healthy, they had massive hidden flaws. Their chromosomes were randomly scattered between the cells of each embryo. Whatever the explanations for this serious barrier to progress with primate clones, it has come as a relief to many groups with ethical concerns over human cloning. Cloning humans may well be impossible, certainly before much more is understood about all the processes involved.

## Designer babies for environmental stress

The possibility of perfect babies, designed to take account of various parental aspirations, or even whims, given the varieties of technological advance just described, has been discussed by some researchers. It is clear, however, that we are unlikely to have the appropriate technology for some time. Nonetheless, there is always the possibility that it might be feasible, some day, to engineer human offspring in such a way as to equip them with extra stress genes that could enable them to survive conditions of very severe environmental hostility. In other words, could they be artificially provided with a set of genes that would allow them to sidestep the time-consuming processes of natural selection in what might be a future environmental situation of dire emergency?

Despite the conceptual attractiveness of genetic engineering techniques to insert stress genes into stress sensitive organisms, thus achieving stress tolerance, progress in this direction may be disappointing. Thus far, our attempts to insert new genes into the chromosomes of victims of inherited diseases in order to replace their defective genes, have been disheartening. However, a real problem is likely to be that many environmental stresses, rather than activating single genes, often result in the activation of several genes. Moreover, several genes are activated by more than one stress. Although we have accumulated considerable knowledge of stress genes and their products, the achievement of stress tolerance in most organisms appears often to involve the complex interaction of many stress gene products.

Notwithstanding these difficulties, some studies have shown that, in certain cases, it is possible to alter the stress tolerance of some organisms by direct gene transfer. For example, fruit flies engineered to carry twelve extra copies of a gene encoding one of the heat shock proteins developed a rapid acquisition of heat tolerance. Plants have also been genetically engineered to resist stress. Tobacco plants, with genes transferred from squash plants for controlling the composition of fats, were found to have an altered sensitivity to low temperatures. Tobacco plants have also been engineered to have an increased tolerance to salt by transferring genes for mannitol production from a type of bacteria. Bacterial genes have been transferred to tobacco plants to increase their resistance to conditions of drought. There have also been examples of the direct transfer of genes from plants in the wild to domesticated varieties of the same family. For instance, a single gene has been taken from a wild rice strain and engineered into a cultivated variety to confer resistance to bacterial blight, which is a considerable hazard to rice growers. How effective such genetically engineered rice varieties will be in the field remains to be seen.

Perhaps most commercial interest has focused on the development of genetically engineered plants resistant to the lethal effects of specific herbicides. Their creation served to signal scientific and public concerns regarding the propagation and environmental release of genetically engineered organisms as a whole. A particularly significant example has been the engineering of resistance to the herbicide glyphosate into commercially important crop species such as soybean and oilseed rape. This was achieved by the transfer of a specific gene from a glyphosate-resistant bacterium to these crops. Unfortunately, due to the nature of its transfer, it was soon discovered that this novel gene could also spread to wild relatives of the crop plants. Not surprisingly, this became a matter of concern to the agricultural industry and environmentalists and also to the public, particularly in the UK. Certainly, problems might well be initiated by gene flow to wild plant relatives, and, more specifically, through the creation of herbicide-tolerant 'super weeds'. Different strategies are now under investigation to circumvent these difficulties, which, understandably, have contributed to the growing public hostility in the UK to genetically engineered crops and their products. This contrasts with a greater public optimism in countries such as the USA, Argentina, Canada and China.

The concept of capitalizing on the discovery of stress genes for the creation of stress-resistant plants has met with limited practical success so far. However, we are still very much at the bottom of the learning curve regarding the activation of stress genes and the interaction of their products in the establishment of tolerances to various stresses. Nonetheless, it may be that the creation of stress-resistant plants is as far as the concept can be pushed. Although animals such as fruit flies can be engineered for heat tolerance, they are quite different from warm-blooded animals. We already have sophisticated physiological systems to provide fairly efficient protection from extremes of temperature. There are, of course, other environmental threats, such as radiation and chemical pollution, which could ultimately threaten our existence. Possibly, with increased levels of antioxidant or detoxifying proteins, we might survive some of these. However, even to equip our cells with the extra genes necessary to make these stress proteins, it will be necessary to improve our gene transfer technology. We have already seen, in the context of gene therapy, that the possibility of efficient and precise transfers of foreign genes into the DNA of egg cells, or embryo cells, remains a remote possibility. Success at this level would be absolutely fundamental to the process of creating human offspring with novel combinations of stress genes. The difficulties with the technology have so far been grossly underestimated, and speculation of future applications leading to designer babies equipped to resist severe environmental stress must remain decidedly premature. On balance, it seems that we are not likely to be able to rush this fence, even if there are those more than eager to do so.

---

### Key points in this chapter

- For some time now we have capitalized on the genes of other species in various ways. To maintain the vigour of most of our staple crop plants, we have regularly plundered the genetic resources of their relatives in the wild using artificial selection.

- The techniques of genetic engineering now enable us to lay siege to millions of years of evolutionary history. We can remove genes from one species and insert them in another, thus producing gene combinations never seen in nature before.

- Gene therapy offers the prospect of using genes as a cure for inherited disease. It involves the replacement of a patient's defective gene with a normal one from another source. However, clinical progress to date has been disappointing, due to a lack of reliable and precise methods.

- Cloning is a new way of making babies. It short-circuits the normal routes of fertilization involving eggs and sperm. So far it has only been carried out with animals such as sheep, cattle, goats and mice. The success rate, however, is poor. There appear to be technical problems that may relate to the equilibrating of adult DNA in the environment of the egg. In many cases, abnormal animal clones have been reported. Despite this, some human cloning has been attempted, though the outcomes remain unpredictable.

- Stress genes have been transferred from one species to another to increase their stress tolerance. Speculation about transferring extra stress genes into human embryos to create offspring more able to tolerate possible future environmental hostilities is premature, however, given the present state of the technology.

# 15

# DNA and planetary stewardship

A mere sixty years ago, we were only just beginning to appreciate that DNA was the key molecule in heredity, but we had no idea what it looked like, or how it operated. Now we understand its stunning simplicity and the miraculous mechanisms by which it is copied and decoded. The recipe of genes that govern the way we are made and how we function has now been elucidated. It is one of the most significant scientific advancements in our history. Whilst many new answers will be forthcoming, these will inevitably raise new questions. We may have thought we were very sophisticated and far removed from other living things, but already we have found that our DNA tells a different story. It seems to be a 'hotchpotch' of genes handed down, albeit with some modifications, from plants, animals and primitive forms of bacteria. We share many genes with flies and worms and, overall, most of our genes are extremely similar to those of other mammals. Indeed, the nucleotide sequences that make up our DNA differ, in general, by only 1.5 per cent from those of chimpanzees. Despite this somewhat deflating information, the general pattern of genes in human DNA is nonetheless unique, and governs our unmatched lifestyle on earth. Our collection of genes is essentially immortal. Individuals may die, but the human blueprint, in its general overall form, will be successively passed from one generation to the next, unless of course there are significant changes to our planetary environment that prevent our continued survival.

The elucidation of the nucleotide sequences that make up the human genome (see Chapter 2) is likely to transform our outlook on the living world and our place in it. A service has recently been offered by Craig Venter, a key player in the work that led to the initial un-ravelling of the human genome (see also Chapter 2), whereby his commercial organization would map, within a week, the genome of any individual prepared to pay in the region of half a million pounds. Such well-heeled individuals would then be offered the possibility of something similar to a CD that would contain the nucleotide sequence of all their own genes, including individual variations and defects.

In the future, personal genetic information is likely to become progressively more readily available. For many, this may raise visions of a 'brave new world', unless safeguards can be put in place that build secure barriers between medical information, employers' records and medical insurance companies. Like it or not, we are now in the midst of a veritable explosion of genetic information. A burgeoning amount of DNA nucleotide sequence information is now readily available on the Internet. Paradoxically, however, some problems are emerging that relate to the 'non-availability' of certain genes. One commercial com-pany already has patents that give it rights over the diagnostic and therapeutic uses of two genes, BRCA-1 and BRCA-2, that have been implicated in the susceptibility to breast and ovarian cancers (see Chapter 10). Essentially this company is in the position of having a monopoly on testing for breast cancer susceptibility genes. Not sur-prisingly, such developments are being challenged and have generated deep animosities within the medical and scientific communities. They perceive acute restrictions on their ability to pursue further academic research related to these particular cancer genes and their biological functions within cells and tissues. In the coming decades, more and more genetic abnormalities associated with human disabilities and diseases are likely to emerge. Patenting that restricts the availability of certain genes raises the spectre of major components of health care falling into the hands of big companies and their legal aides.

## Planetary stewardship

A look into the night sky, with its glittering points of light, reminds us that we are ephemeral, contingent parts of a silent universe that is vastly larger than ourselves. The last century saw dramatic progress towards a greater scientific understanding of the universe and the deepest mysteries of its creation. Everything we have learnt since the days of Galileo indicates that nebulas and galaxies are completely indifferent to our fate. The universe seems eternally silent and its scale is massively beyond our comprehension. It has been estimated that there are as many as 50 billion galaxies, and even within our own galaxy there may be 100 billion stars. From DNA studies we will undoubtedly gain some clearer ideas of our origin and evolution on this planet over the last 4 billion years, but cosmological studies indicate that the universe is much older. From the age of the oldest stars it is now hypothesized that the universe evolved from a Big Bang 15 billion years ago. The chemistry of our bodies shows clearly that we are made from the same set of elements as stars. Every atom in each of us, with the exception of hydrogen, was originally created by the nuclear fusion events within stars of the Milky Way, even before the sun or earth was created. As generations of stars were created and subsequently died, the quantities of elements like carbon, nitrogen and oxygen increased, so that by 5 billion years ago, when the solar system was condensed by gravity, it contained a significant proportion of this detritus of long-deceased stars. Chemically, we are little different from the rest of the universe.

Although we now are beginning to appreciate our origins and what we are made of, and that we are contingent parts of a universe vastly larger than ourselves, questions remain that relate to our future. On the face of it, our planet will continue to exist for a long time to come. Estimates suggest that the sun has another fifteen billion years before it burns out. However, 15 billion years is a time beyond human comprehension, and many critical changes could take place on the earth in the more immediate future. We have to accept that this planet, and the diversity of its life forms, are our responsibility and ours alone. The cosmos exists independently of ourselves and, from current scientific evidence, is completely oblivious as to how we manage our local planetary environment. We must shoulder the responsibility for being alive at this particular moment in the history of our planet; we owe it to future generations. Our activities are undoubtedly changing the earth's environment, and our genes and those of other species are under siege and suffering as a result. There is an urgent need to develop a sense of planetary stewardship: the job needs to be done and there is no one else to do it, unless you believe in a listening and interventionist god.

## We depend on the diversity of life forms

There have been a number of recent attempts to estimate the number of species of living organisms that share the earth with us. Although around 1.5 to 1.8 million distinct species have already been described, it may be that the total lies somewhere in the region of 5 million. This may even be a conservative estimate; as many as 30 million have been suggested. This represents a vast library of genes upon which, in theory, we could draw, with our new expertise in genetic engineering. There could well be potentially useful stress-avoiding genes that could be used as a lifebelt, if environmental conditions threaten our existence.

Efforts are also being made to evaluate the likely rates of species extinction. Alarming figures of around 4,000 to 14,000 lost per year are being suggested. In contrast, when the fossil record is examined, although the majority of species that have ever existed on earth are now extinct, there would appear to be a background extinction rate of one to five species per year. On this basis, species are now being lost at a rate that is many times more rapid than at any previous time in the earth's history. These extinctions seriously diminish the planetary gene bank. Mankind is the primary driving force behind these extinctions, through efforts to modify the natural environment to create new land for agriculture, industry and dwellings. However, it is only recently that the value and magnitude of biodiversity have been fully appreciated. We are heavily dependent on the biodiversity of living species for a variety of essential services, including the recycling of atmospheric gases (such as carbon dioxide and oxygen), water and nutrients. It has been argued that biodiversity is our least appreciated resource. It provides a basis for food, medicines, shelter and clothing. The rapidly increasing list of extinct species makes our attempts to engineer a stable genetic future a more doubtful prospect.

Mankind's ability to alter the landscape drastically distinguishes us from most other species. It has been estimated that roughly a quarter of the carbon dioxide in the atmosphere at the moment is the result of the transformation of tropical forests into pasturelands. Tropical forest systems are important for the maintenance of acceptable atmospheric levels of carbon dioxide. As the level of atmospheric carbon dioxide increases, a greenhouse effect is produced, which could have long-term effects on global climate, profoundly altering the weather conditions across different regions of the world. Plant and animal populations, if they are unable to migrate rapidly enough to survive, will have to adapt to new conditions as they arise in their particular geographic region. Natural selection is likely to propel these populations in the direction of appropriate adaptation, but, if the climatic change is too abrupt, adaptation may be beyond the limits of these selective mechanisms. Unfortunately, such adjustments operate over long timescales. Overall, the effectiveness and survival capability of a population will depend on its level of genetic variability. In the event, the species that are best able to deal with climatic changes are those that can both migrate and adapt. They will have large populations spread over wide geographical areas. In contrast, climatic changes induced by global warming may well present considerable threats to the survival of small populations of endangered species. Five times in the past history of our planet, environmental conditions changed to such an extent that most of the life forms became extinct. At least one of these mass extinctions was most likely caused by extreme environmental change subsequent to the impact of a massive meteorite. Today, the earth may well be in the middle of a sixth extinction, triggered not by any external influence, but by man's destructive ways.

## Is a less toxic future possible?

Even if we cannot turn the clock back two hundred years or so, a question posed by Sandra Steingraber in her book *Living Downstream* is, 'Can we do anything that might ensure a less toxic future for ourselves and other species on Earth?' It is one thing finding out why our environment is changing for the worse. It is quite another matter to find ways of dealing with the situation. Most of the problems do not recognize national borders. Solutions require agreement from many competing interests, national and economic, but domestic politics and the likelihood of national economic privations, such as unemployment, can readily put the brakes on progress.

### The threat of nuclear radiation

Atmospheric testing of nuclear weapons is a thing of the past. However, the question remains: is nuclear radiation still a threat to our genes and general well-being? In many respects, the nuclear issue has almost disappeared from public consciousness. On a global scale, it is fair to say that the number of cancer deaths specifically attributable to nuclear radiation is extremely small. Most DNA damage and cancer deaths from radiation today can be blamed on excessive exposure to UVB rays from the sun. Many countries have lost their enthusiasm for nuclear power, but it is still a dangerous technology. As recently as 1999 there was a serious incident at a uranium fuel production plant at Tokaimura in Japan. Such accidents mean that we should not be complacent about our safety, especially in view of the real uncertainties regarding what constitutes a safe dose of radiation. In 1958 there was a serious fire in the power plant at Windscale, UK; in 1979 there was a core meltdown at Three Mile Island in the USA; and in 1986 a serious explosion occurred at Chernobyl in the Ukraine. All these had serious health consequences, not only for those living in the vicinity but also for many at considerable distances. There is still governmental support in some countries for continuing with nuclear power. Although relatively few new reactors are now being built, these are mainly in developing countries. A more general policy has been to extend the life of old reactors, with all the doubts that such procedures conjure up. Whatever safety standards are imposed, there are still question marks hanging over the use of nuclear power. On the credit side, nuclear reactors do not burn fossil fuel and have been suggested as a means of escape from global warming. To foster a new lease of life for the nuclear industry on this basis would simply divert us from the more urgent task of developing other technologies to meet our power requirements that do not contribute to global warming or generate hazardous waste. The nuclear industry has yet to demonstrate convincingly that it can deal with the highly dangerous radioactive wastes that are an inevitable consequence of the nuclear fuel cycle. Nuclear reprocessing still accounts for the majority of radioactive leaks into the atmosphere and surrounding waters. Moreover, a satisfactory explanation for the apparently high rate of leukaemias suffered by children in the vicinity of some plants is anxiously awaited. One survey suggested that this might be linked to the radiation to which fathers had been exposed whilst working in the plants. This view has been vigorously contested, but is nevertheless a symptom of serious public concern.

Clear signs exist that nuclear power may well have had its day, at least in the UK. There is now more real pressure at government level to consider renewable energy as an effective way of reducing future carbon dioxide emissions. It is envisaged that this could be achieved by expanding the number of wind turbines on land and offshore and by utilizing wave power and underwater tidal generators. Hopefully, these renewable sources of energy will be allowed to prosper and so contribute significantly to our power requirements.

## Ozone destroyers

Chemicals that destroy atmospheric ozone continue to increase worldwide. CFC molecules released at ground level can take many years to reach the stratosphere. Even when degraded to chlorine, each atom has a very considerable lifespan and can destroy many thousands of stratospheric ozone molecules. It may be that reductions in the worldwide releases of CFCs, even if immediate, may not be rapid enough to protect our genes, and those of other life forms on earth, from the serious hazards of much increased UVB radiation.

Fourteen years ago, the governments of the world agreed in Montreal to phase out the manufacture of CFCs and halons responsible for most of the damage to the ozone layer in the stratosphere (see Chapter 8). By 1996, many industrialized countries had banned most uses of these chemicals. Russia will shortly come into line, but China has been permitted a ten-year respite. Some financial aid from Western governments may well be required to ensure appropriate phasing-out programmes. The route to ozone recovery will involve intense diplomatic effort among the participants in the Montreal Protocol to elicit the necessary level of global stewardship. Inevitably, this will sometimes present local difficulties. For example, in the UK, because of uncertainties surrounding the interpretation of a 1998 EU directive, delays have arisen over the disposal of old refrigerators. The directive issued guidelines to cut down on European emissions of ozone-destroying gases from discarded fridges, which now must be destroyed in expensive recycling plants. As a result, it was estimated that the UK could face a bill for £75 million as a 'fridge mountain' grew at the rate of 6,500 a day, piling up in disused hangars and warehouses, with many being dumped by the roadside. There have been recent suggestions that newer disposal procedures may alleviate the problem.

## The menacing chemical environment

The menace from our chemical environment most readily impinges on our consciousness when spectacular accidents occur. Such a major disaster occurred in 1984 at a Union Carbide plant in Bhopal, India, which resulted in the massive release of *methyl isocyanate* – produced for use in the production of pesticides, polyurethane foam and plastics – and some hydrogen cyanide. Between 4,000 and 8,000 people died at the time, and the overall death toll has been estimated at over 20,000. At least 120,000 people continue to have severe medical problems, including eye and respiratory problems, reproductive difficulties and birth defects, and some cancers. While eyes and lungs are the primary targets for methyl isocyanate, there is evidence that it may also affect fetal development. However, despite the reported incidence of cancers, there is yet no firm basis to account for this, such as a specific inter-action with DNA, or cancer genes.

More generally, the years since 1945 have seen a massive increase in the rate at which novel synthetic chemicals have been created. It has been estimated that there are now around 75,000 in common use, many of which are a serious threat to genes, and against which we have no natural protection. In the workplace, much protective legislation has been evolved but unfortunately it is not just industrial workers that are risk. Many of these chemicals are now produced in such massive amounts that they are no longer confined to the workplace, but slowly seep into the environment due to their release into air and water as toxic wastes, accidental spills or runoff from farmland. Many environ-mental carcinogens find their way into our food. Indeed, low levels of some of these could now be viewed as basic contaminants. Although in some cases, like DDT and PCBs, bans on their use in the USA, and in many other countries, came into operation in the 1970s, it is still possible to detect traces of these compounds, or substances derived from them, that have accumulated in human tissues.

Unfortunately in the process of prohibiting the use of DDT, we may have deprived ourselves of perhaps the cheapest and most effective weapon in the fight against malaria. Many therapies are now available to combat a variety of mosquito-borne diseases. Despite this, the insect and the pathogens that it carries have proven to be hardy, cunning and remorseless. Mosquitoes and their associated diseases are still very much a threat worldwide. Indeed things seem to be getting worse, with millions of deaths every year. The tropics are now plagued with drug-resistant malaria. Regions of the planet previously thought to be clear of malaria are being hit once again. No other chemical is as potent as DDT against the resting mosquito. It has a considerable number of advantages. It can be used as first line of attack, and despite the fact that mosquitoes can develop resistance following DDT exposure, this does not affect their susceptibility to other more costly insecticides. In 2000, although the use of DDT is virtually prohibited worldwide, under a UN Environmental Programme Treaty, a stay of execution was granted. It is still manufactured in India and China with the strict understanding that it is to be used solely in anti-malaria programmes. Despite the undoubted health risks already discussed, this move may yet be crucial in the increasingly difficult crusade against the ravages of malaria. Mosquitoes are still probably our deadliest foe and certainly do not appear on the list of currently endangered species – far from it!

In general, while consumption of natural carcinogens known to be present in food is likely to have remained unchanged over the last fifty years, the presence of small amounts of synthetic carcinogens arising from air and water is likely to continue increasing. There is an urgent need for vigilance and awareness of the increasing hazards of synthetic chemicals in the environment. Many complex issues are involved. Our knowledge of gene action, DNA damage and the development of various cancers, whilst increasing rapidly, is as yet insufficient to provide a convincing basis for foolproof testing. Indeed, we are confronted not just by single chemicals, but by more and more complex cocktails of hazardous substances. This seriously limits the effectiveness of any predictive testing. Because avoidance is not a simple matter, like dodging DNA-damaging cigarette smoke, some long-term strategy for chemical hazards in the environment is essential. Although we could limit their use, our present lifestyles, at least in Western nations, will make this difficult both economically and politically. Certainly, we can readily ban the use of those chemicals that are clearly proven dangerous. However, as has been the case for CFCs, this may take time, effort and money to enforce worldwide. Some substances may leave a fatal legacy, even although their further use is severely curtailed, as was the case with DDT and PCBs. This is because the rate at which they are broken down in the environment is extremely slow. A possible route out of these difficulties may be to give serious consideration to cleaning up the environment using microbes or plants.

## Microbial genes to the rescue

*Bioremediation* refers to the general processes whereby some microbes and plants can act on pollutants to remedy, or eliminate, environmental pollution. This includes the reduction of the chemical waste content of soils, ground water and effluents from food processing and chemical plants. In its simplest form, bioremediation relies on the array of microbes normally resident in soils or ground water. The assumption is made that the microorganisms at the site are already adapted to the particular chemical wastes, and can break these down, provided they are adequately supplied with oxygen, nitrates and phosphates.

Due to their versatility, microorganisms play a particularly fundamental role in the global recycling of matter. They excel at utilizing natural or synthetic chemicals for their nutrition and energy requirements. They have coexisted with an immense variety of chemical compounds for billions of years. Together with the compounds that make up the bodies of living organisms, the natural world contains a diversity of chemicals produced by living organisms, as well as chemical compounds such as those in coal, petroleum and natural gas production, created by geological processes. Petroleum oils originate from the accumulation of phytoplankton residues in ancient shallow seas; whilst they are complex, they mainly comprise paraffins, cycloparaffins and aromatics such as benzene. Coal, on the other hand, is mainly derived from fossilized terrestrial plant matter and is made up of complex aromatic and polycyclic structures. It also contains a variety of sulphur compounds. Over many years, sources like these have provided microorganisms with a vast diversity of substances for their nourishment and growth. This has resulted in the evolution of genes encoding proteins capable of breaking down widely disparate natural chemicals using a variety of routes. Such a repository of genes now serves as a platform for further evolutionary steps to permit the microorganisms of soils and water to break down new synthetic compounds as they arise in the environment, due to human activity.

Natural microbial communities are complex groups of highly inter-dependent microorganisms. Chemical compounds are usually more effectively degraded in environments containing an array of micro-organisms, rather than single organisms, since the range of breakdown possibilities is likely to be greater in a community. Products created by one microorganism in the community during the breakdown of a chemical compound are quite likely to be taken up by others, so that the process of degradation can be continued. Overall, the combined activity of several organisms is likely to lead to the complete degrada-tion of the contaminant to carbon dioxide, water and minerals.

An important application of this microbial versatility can be seen in present-day treatment of sewage and wastewater. This exploits the degradative capabilities of various bacteria and fungi to remove organic matter. A class of soil bacteria, *Pseudomonads*, utilizes a wide range of compounds as nutrition and energy sources. Many of these com-pounds are broken down by proteins that are, in fact, encoded not by genes in the main chromosomes of these bacteria, but by genes carried on *plasmids*. These are small circular DNA molecules that normally exist within bacteria, but that are copied independently of the main bacterial chromosome. Some plasmids are relatively small and carry only one or two genes, while others can be up to a fifth of the size of the main chromosome. An important attribute is that plasmids can be transferred from one bacterium to another. There are many groups of *Pseudomonads* in soil, each carrying a distinct plasmid carrying the genes for proteins to break down a certain type of chemical com-pound. As these plasmids are transmissible between the different groups of *Pseudomonads*, there is the potential for the exploitation of a wide range of degradative possibilities of potentially toxic chemical compounds, through what can be viewed as a highly effective form of gene sharing.

Microorganisms can break down an enormous range of chemical compounds originating from natural biological and geological pro-cesses. However, many synthetic compounds, released into the environ-ment from industrial and agricultural sources, have no clear relationship with compounds already in the natural world. Such chemicals are often referred to as xenobiotics. In many cases, these can remain unchanged in the environment for considerable periods of time. They include halogenated aliphatic and aromatic compounds, phthalate esters and polycyclic aromatic hydrocarbons, many of which are distributed as components of fertilizers, herbicides and pesticides. Others, such as dioxins, furans and polycyclic aromatic hydrocarbons, arise from incinerators and can also be detected in waste effluents as a result of the production and use of synthetic products. A hazardous aspect of these xenobiotics is that they can become progressively more concentrated with each step in the food chain. Striking examples are PCBs (polychlorinated biphenyls) and phthalate esters (plasticizers for cellulose and vinyl plastics), which can act as hormone mimics disrupting the normal activities of key animal and human sex hormones (see Chapter 11). PCBs have a wide range of applications, including hydraulic fluids, plasticizers, lubricants, flame retardants and dielectric fluids; although their manufacture was halted in 1977, their breakdown in the environment has been excruciatingly slow.

Since there is already an enormous range of microorganisms capable of breaking down a variety of environmental chemicals, a reasonable question now is whether the new techniques of genetic engineering can be used to improve the prospects of pollution control. In principle at least, it would be possible to create in one microorganism an assemblage of hand-picked genes, originally from disparate bacterial species that encode proteins specifically capable of breaking down pollutants hitherto difficult to deal with. Many environmentalists, however, are likely to look askance at the thought of releasing such a genetically engineered organism into the soil and public acceptance might be hard to achieve. In reality such an engineered 'super-bug' may have only a limited capacity for survival in the real environment, as distinct from the relatively cosseted surroundings of the laboratory. It would have to face potentially novel, and possibly hostile, conditions as well as intensive competition from bacteria already thriving in the soil. Despite these potential difficulties, there have been recent field trials in the USA of the bacterium *Pseudomanas fluorescens*, genetically engineered to break up toxic hydrocarbons such as naphthalene and anthracene. Over a two-year period, the naphthalene content of the contaminated soil used in the trial did decrease, but whether this was due to the engineered bacteria or to microorganisms already present in the soil was not clear. In any event, the genetically engineered bacteria remained in the soil and none was detected in the drainage water. While this might allay some of the concerns of environmentalists, there is still the possibility of transfer of genes from the engineered bacteria to those occurring naturally in the soil, with consequences difficult to predict.

A different approach to soil remediation being explored at present is the use of plants. *Phytoremediation* capitalizes on the properties of plants able to survive in contaminated soils and water. A number of plants are able to absorb high levels of contaminants with their roots and concentrate them there, or in their leaves or shoots. Usually such plant species are found in areas where the soil contains greater than normal amounts of toxic metals, as a result of pollution or geological factors. Alpine pennycress is especially effective at accumulating zinc, cadmium or lead. *Assylum* species, which accumulate nickel, have already been used in soil bioremediation field trials, and plants from many other families have also been shown to remove cobalt, copper, chromium, manganese or selenium from contaminated soils. The ideal plants should be able to accumulate several different metals and function effectively even when the environmental concentration is relatively low, as well as being resistant to diseases and pests. Whether plants can be effectively used in the bioremediation of soils and water contaminated with xenobiotics is presently under investigation. In addition, some plants have been genetically engineered to contain genes from bacterial species that also might facilitate this type of bioremediation.

## Can we cure cancer?

Progress towards a less toxic future looks like being a slow business, even if cooperation on a worldwide scale can be achieved. An increased incidence of cancer is a significant reality of our present environmental predicament. For some clinicians, the best cure for cancer is its early detection. An even better solution might be to make lifestyle choices that would drastically reduce the chances of gene damage and the development of cancer. Evading exposure to direct sunlight, avoiding inhaling tobacco smoke or automobile exhaust fumes, keeping away from the vicinity of nuclear power or reprocessing plants, and eating plenty of fruits and vegetables would seem to be a good start, but, as already pointed out, many environmental agents which can damage DNA and may act as carcinogens are much more difficult to avoid. Epidemiologists have attempted to grade the overall severity of risk to put these issues in some general perspective. We now know that well over a third of all cancer deaths can be linked to tobacco smoke. It is by far the major atmospheric carcinogen. One could almost be forgiven for not taking environmental advice from anyone who smokes. By comparison, the risks from radiation are extremely small, despite contemporary worries to the contrary. At this time only 2 per cent of cancers in the USA are specifically attributable to radiation, and the bulk of these are caused by radiation from the sun, rather than any exposure to radioactivity.

Our diet constitutes another risk. The proportion of cancer deaths due to diet has been estimated by some as equivalent to that caused by tobacco smoke. However, this is a complex issue clouded with uncertainties and it seems that overeating and lack of exercise may also contribute to the risks of acquiring certain cancers. As our foodstuffs contain many thousands of different chemicals, both natural and synthetic, some of which are known to be carcinogenic in experimental animals, it is extremely difficult to be specific with regard to risk. Furthermore, many environmental carcinogens readily enter the food chain and can concentrate progressively in the fatty tissues of animals we eat. It is therefore not surprising that links have been suggested between colon and rectal cancer and dietary animal fat. Fat-rich diets are also believed to contribute to breast cancer.

What can be done to clarify these serious uncertainties, so that people can be authoritatively advised on how to minimize the risks? More testing is a constant plea, but this can only make sense if it can be carried out on the basis of a firmer understanding of the intricate mechanisms that contribute to the development of different cancers. Although spectacular advances have been made in respect of the genetic basis of cancer progression, and the role of mutations in the processes, questions remain regarding the precise causes of specific cancers and the possible role of environmental chemicals. The role of hormones in cancers of the breast, cervix, ovaries and prostate also comprises another area of uncertainty. Because of this, a proper evaluation of the carcinogenic hazards of hormone mimics and disrupters is fraught with difficulties at present. Solid evidence is now urgently required to assist in the development of more informative tests. Too often our acquisition of understanding has been slow. By the time the hazards of a particular environmental chemical are understood, the process of tumour development in individuals previously exposed may well be very far advanced.

Of all medical investigations, research into cancer is particularly well supported both by charities and by government agencies. Sometimes the focus of this research has been the subject of criticism. Should more effort be put into finding expensive drug-based cures, when there is considerable evidence that a significant number of cancers can be avoided by judicious lifestyle choices? Should more resources be put into preventative strategies, or into improving patient care? Rightly, a great deal of present cancer research aims to achieve a fundamental understanding of the basic mechanisms that govern cell behaviour leading to the development of various major cancers. The possibility of more meaningful tests and a much clearer evaluation of the possible risks are likely to emerge from this systematic approach. These will enhance the credibility of future preventative strategies. Accurate evaluation of the basic mechanisms of cancer development also has the advantage that it will provide a firmer platform for the rational development of specific anticancer drugs. In Chapter 11, the history of some early anticancer drugs was described. A basic property of these was their ability to damage DNA and thereby interfere with the processes of correct DNA copying prior to cell division. The problem is that, although they reduce the proliferation of cancer cells, they are unspecific. As well as reducing the proliferation of cancers cells, many also interfere with the proliferation of important normal cells in the body. Many of these drugs are still in current use; among other things, they seriously weaken a patient's immune system. Furthermore, other toxic effects make patients feel tired and unwell. In short, chemotherapy, as used at the moment, is a blunt instrument, with many undesirable clinical side effects due to the lack of specificity. In light of these experiences, the search for cancer cures sometimes seems like the search for the Holy Grail. Steady progress towards a greater understanding of cancer development may well provide a sounder basis for the development of new drugs with the desired selectivity towards cancer cells.

One such example has been the growing appreciation of the role of the protein p53, which is now a promising candidate for exploitation in the search for a cancer cure. Mutations in the gene encoding this protein are very common, having been detected in over half of all types of human cancer. This gene is now perhaps the most widely researched in history. As previously described, its product, the p53 protein, normally plays a key role as an emergency brake on cell division. Mutations in its gene, however, can result in defective versions of the protein that can set cells free of the normal restraints on their proliferation. This is one of the hallmarks of cancer cells. Sir David Lane, a biochemist in Dundee, and one of the discoverers of p53, has recently instigated the design of drugs that will reactivate the defective p53 protein in cancer cells. The beauty of this approach is that it should specifically switch off the proliferation of cancer cells, as distinct from normal cells. Knowledge of the precise structure of the p53 protein has been patiently acquired over the past few years and has enabled computers to aid in the precise design of such novel activator drugs. Clinical tests with one of these activator drugs on terminally ill patients with head and neck cancers suggest that this is a promising approach. In addition to these developments involving p53, there are many research groups around the world using different approaches, but all attempting to create drugs that will specifically target tumour cells.

The potential availability of specific anticancer drugs in the not too distant future is likely to raise other complex issues. The dangers of tobacco smoking are now well known, but many smokers seem unable to stop. Should we be pressurized into making more sensible lifestyle choices and made to pay for the consequences if we don't? Thus far, pressure through increased taxes on tobacco and widespread advertising on the dangers has had only limited effects.

## Stewardship

Arguments about the use and costs of drugs as quick-fix cures for cancers produced by lifestyle choices that put our suffering genes under siege reflect, at a personal level, some of the larger issues that now concern the well-being of our planet. For instance, how can individual countries, in the interest of the planet, be persuaded to adopt different lifestyles with regard to greenhouse gas emissions or release of ozone-destroying CFCs? At least there is a declining enthusiasm for nuclear power, balanced by an apparently genuine interest at government levels in the possibilities of developing alternative sources of energy. To speed this up, there may need to be higher taxation or economic sanctions to help reduce our reliance on fossil fuels, even though this could create economic and social problems in the short term. Overall, it is likely that the richer nations will not only have to set standards of behaviour but also provide monetary assistance to enable poorer countries achieve these standards without crippling financial and social hardship.

In this context, it is worth very briefly summarizing the political progress that has occurred over the last decade. In 1992 the UN sponsored an *Earth Summit* in Rio de Janeiro. Its general aim was to serve as a focus for international political attention and certainly there was a spirit of optimism and promises of cooperation.

Agenda 21, which laid out in forty chapters what was essentially a 'blueprint' for the twenty-first century, was produced. A *Framework Convention on Climate Change* gathered 170 signatories to slash their greenhouse gas emissions back to 1990 levels by 2002. The *Kyoto Protocol* later strengthened this in 1997. It sought to control countries, by legal means, to further reductions so as to cut levels to 6–8 per cent below those of 1990 by 2012. Additionally a *Biodiversity Convention* attracted 180 international signatories. The general objective was to ensure benefits from resources such as drugs from tropical plants are distributed equably between those parties concerned. There was also a *Biosafety Protocol* that gives countries the right to veto the import of genetically engineered organisms.

Despite the lofty promises, progress has been disappointing. By 2002 only Denmark has increased its contribution to developing countries. The contribution, as a percentage of GNP, from the UK has remained static, while the contributions from France, Canada and the USA have been considerably reduced. Basically, rich countries have continued to champion free trade in the belief that free markets will produce the enabling scientific discoveries that will lead to appropriate solutions. Unfortunately, free trade is still leading to the further erosion of the environmental resources, such as the forests of poor countries, bringing increasing conflict with the aims of biodiversity and biosafety. Only seventy countries at this time have national conservation strategies. Minimal prices are still being paid for valuable timber resources, and in the past decade around 4 per cent of the world's forests have been lost. The environment of poor countries is still under extraordinary attack.

In terms of greenhouse gas emissions, there has been a 9.1 per cent *increase* each year in the last decade. Although EU countries have reduced their emissions, Australia and the USA have increased theirs by over 20 per cent. While the Kyoto Protocol was endorsed by President Clinton, his successor, President Bush, subsequently backed out.

Possibly to stimulate flagging resolve in the years that followed the Earth Summit in Rio de Janeiro, a *World Summit on Sustainable Development* was convened in Johannesburg in 2002. The aim was to promote the fight against poverty and protection of the environment. Crucial areas focused on were water, energy, health, agriculture and biodiversity. However, in the event, nothing that was agreed was obligatory. There was nevertheless general agreement to diminish the environmental impacts of chemicals by 2020, but there were no specific targets for renewable energy, merely an invitation to countries to build up their outputs from wind farms and solar power 'with a sense of urgency'. In terms of biodiversity, the deal to reduce the current rate of species loss by 2010 seemed to lack any teeth.

The general notion at Johannesburg that governments should 'promote corporate responsibility and accountability' was all very reasonable, as was the pledge to confront overconsumption by rich countries. Nonetheless, the business of policing all these agreements, which is crucial, is to remain within the remit of the 'Commission for Sustainable Development', a body originally set up by the UN to oversee the implementation of 'Agenda 21', which emerged from the Rio Summit ten years before. At this moment in earth's history, despite significant political efforts, pollution is still on the increase, valuable natural resources are still being pillaged, and the gap between rich and poor still widens.

Political attempts to solve our environmental ills seem to have become routed into the slow lane. Basically, it falls to us alone to look after our planet, as we are the only species that understands the issues confronting the survival of present life forms. There is no one to bail us out, nor are there any quick fixes. Stewardship of the planet and all its life forms is now our collective responsibility; without it, we, and all other life forms, may have to pay a heavy price. Unity with nature is the foundation of our existence on this planet. Along with all living organisms, we do not simply confront an autonomous physical world. Together we make a significant contribution to the assembly of the environment: we cannot live without changing it. Because of our particular genetic make-up, we have the power to change the world more rapidly and more comprehensively than other organisms. Our lifestyles are now such that we could easily re-create the environment in a way that is potentially hostile to our continued survival. It could be argued that it is *our own genes*, by influencing our make-up and behaviour, that are contributing to the present restructuring of the environment.

The DNA of our genes may be suffering, but our genes are also at the root of the problem. Nevertheless, it is our genes that give us the potential to solve our present difficulties.

---

**Key points in this chapter**

- Current scientific evidence indicates that the cosmos is completely oblivious to how we manage our planetary environment. It is our responsibility alone.

- We are undoubtedly changing the earth's environment, and our genes are coming under siege. Genes are essentially immortal, as they are passed from one generation to the next. They are the key to our health and well-being, as well as to our continued presence on earth.

- The biodiversity of life forms represent an invaluable gene library. Extinctions will reduce the scope of this genetic resource and may prejudice attempts to engineer a stable genetic future.

- Efforts must be made to create a less toxic future. These will need international cooperation and must include: reducing the release of ozone-destroying chemicals; exploring and utilizing alternative sources of renewable energy rather than relying on fossil fuels or nuclear power; and, particularly, tackling the problem of increasing hazards of synthetic chemicals in the environment.
- Genes from microbes offer potential future rescue routes in the clean-up of chemically contaminated environmental sites. Genes encoding proteins that can break down xenobiotic chemicals, and detoxify poisonous metals, are particularly important.
- Sensible lifestyle choices could reduce the chances of environmentally caused gene damage and the development of cancer. Nevertheless, some drugs are being developed that offer the promise of possible cancer cures.
- Stewardship of the planet and all its life forms is now our collective responsibility; without it we, and all other life forms, may have to pay a heavy price. Our genes, by influencing our make-up and behaviour, are contributing to the present restructuring of the environment.

# References

## Chapter 1

Asma, S., 2001, *Stuffed Animals and Pickled Heads: The Culture and Evolution of Natural History Museums*, Oxford: Oxford University Press.

Barber, L., 1980, *The Heyday of Natural History: 1820–1870*, New York: Doubleday.

Brash, D.E., 1997, Sunlight and the onset of skin cancer, *Trends in Genetics* 13: 410–14.

Bryson, B., 2001, *Down Under*, London: Black Swan.

Bowman, W. C. and Rand, M.J., 1980, *Textbook of Pharmacology* 2nd edn, Oxford: Blackwell Scientific.

Clark, M., 1986, *A Short History of Australia*, Ringwood, VA: Penguin Books.

Christie, M., 2000, *The Ozone Layer*, Cambridge: Cambridge University Press.

Garfield, S., 2000, *Mauve: How One Man Invented a Colour that Changed the World*, London: Faber & Faber.

Hough, R., 1994, *Captain Cook: A Biography*, London: Hodder & Stoughton.

Lakhani, S.R., Dilly, S.A. and Finlayson, C.J., 1993, *Basic Pathology: An Introduction to the Mechanisms of Disease*, London: Edward Arnold.

Leffell, D.J. and Brash, D.E., 1996, Sunlight and skin cancer, *Scientific American* 275, July: 38–43.

Porter, R., 1997, *The Greatest Benefit to Mankind: A Medical History of Humanity from Antiquity to the Present*, London: HarperCollins.

Venzmer, G., 1972, *5000 Years of Medicine*, London: MacDonald.

Wingard, L.B., Brody, T.M., Larner, J. and Schwartz, A., 1991, *Human Pharmacology: Molecular to Clinical*, London: Wolfe Publishing.

## Chapter 2

Alberts, B., Johnson, A., Lewis, J., Raff, M., Roberts, K. and Walter, P., 2002, *Molecular Biology of the Cell*, 4th edn, New York: Garland.

Bolshover, S.R., Hyams, J.S., Jones, S., Shepherd, E.A. and White, H.A., 1997, *From Genes to Cells*, New York: Wiley–Liss.

Coen, E., 1997, *The Art of Genes: How Organisms Make Themselves*, Oxford: Oxford University Press.

Davies, K., 2000, *Cracking the Genome: Inside the Race to Unlock Human DNA*, New York: Free Press.

Davies, K, 2001, *The Sequence: Inside the Race for the Human Genome*, London: Weidenfeld & Nicolson.

Garfield, S., 2000, *Mauve: How One Man Invented a Colour that Changed the World*, London: Faber & Faber.

Griffiths, A.J.F., Miller, J.H., Susuki, D.T., Lewontin, R.C. and Gelbart, W.M., 1996, *An Introduction to Genetic Analysis* 6th edn, New York: W.H. Freeman.

Hartl, D.L. and Jones, E.W., 1998, *Genetics: Principles and Analysis*, 4th edn, Sudbury, MA: Jones & Bartlett.

Henig, R.M., 2000, *A Monk and Two Peas: The Story of Gregor Mendel and the Discovery of Genetics*, London: Weidenfeld & Nicolson.

Karp, G., 1996, *Cell and Molecular Biology: Concepts and Experiments*, New York: John Wiley.

Lodish, H., Berk, A., Zipursky, S.L., Matsudaira, P., Baltimore, D. and Darnell, J., 2000, *Molecular Cell Biology*, 4th edn, New York: W.H. Freeman.

Mange, E.J. and Mange, A.P., 1994, *Basic Human Genetics*, Sunderland, MA: Sinauer Associates.

McConkey, E.H., 1993, *Human Genetics*, Boston: Jones & Bartlett.

Watson, J.D., 1970, *The Double Helix: A Personal Account of the Discovery of the Structure of DNA*, Harmondsworth: Penguin.

Weiner, J., 1999, *Time, Love, Memory: A Great Biologist and the Quest for the Origins of Behaviour*, London: Faber & Faber.

Wolfe, S.L., 1993, *Molecular and Cell Biology*, Belmont, CA: Wadsworth.

## Chapter 3

Alper, T., 1979, *Cellular Radiobiology*, Cambridge: Cambridge University Press.

Bunyard, P., 1999, It couldn't happen here, *The Ecologist* 29: 402–7.

Bunyard, P. and Poche, P., 1999, Nuclear power: time to end the experiment, *The Ecologist* 29: 386–9.

Busby, C., 1999, Poisoning in the name of progress, *The Ecologist* 29: 395–401.

Edwards, R., 1997, Radiation roulette, *New Scientist*, 11 October: 37–40.

Frieberg, E.C., Walker, G.C. and Siede, W., 1995, *DNA Repair and Mutagenesis*, Washington DC: ASM Press.

Gaines, M., 2000, Radiation risk, *New Scientist*, 18 March, Inside Science No. 129.

Hartl, D.L. and Jones, E.W., 1998, *Genetics: Principles and Analysis*, 4th edn, Sudbury, MA: Jones & Bartlett.

Halliwell, B. and Aruoma, O.I., 1993, *DNA and Free Radicals*, New York: Ellis Harwood.
Henry, M., 1999, The woman who knew too much, *The Ecologist* 29: 404–5.
Lawrence, C.W., 1971, *Cellular Radiobiology*, London: Edward Arnold.
Quinn, S., 1995, *Marie Curie: A Life*, London: William Heinemann.
Taylor, A.J.P., 1976, *The Second World War*, Harmondsworth: Penguin Books.

## Chapter 4

British Association and Royal Society of Edinburgh, 2001, *Good to Talk? Mobile Phone Technology,* Report 19, London: British Association.
Busby, C., 2000, And the dangers pylon, *The Ecologist*, 30: 50.
Concar, D., Graham-Rowe, D. and Marks, P. 1999, Special investigation: mobile phones, *New Scientist*, 10 April: 20–25.
Day, M. and Kleiner, K, 1999, Mixed Messages, *New Scientist*, 29 May: 5.
Gibson, I., 1999, Mobile phones under investigation, *Biologist* 46: 147.
Graham-Rowe, D., 2002, Wake-up call, *New Scientist*, 9 February: 4–5.
Department of Health, 2001, *Mobile Phones and Health*, London: DOH.
International Expert Group on Mobile Phones, 'The Stewart Group', 2000, *Expert Group Report: Mobile Phones and Health*, Didcot: National Radiological Protection Board, Didcot
Repacholi, M.H. and Ahlbom, A., 1999, Link between electromagnetic fields and childhood cancer unresolved, *Lancet* 354: 1918–19.
UK Childhood Cancer Study Investigators, 1999, Exposure to power-frequency magnetic fields and the risk of childhood cancer, *Lancet* 354: 1925–31.

## Chapter 5

Alleman, J.E. and Mossman, B.T., 1997, Asbestos revisited, *Scientific American*, July: 54–57.
Ames, B.N. and Gold, L.S., 1997, Environmental pollution, pesticides and the prevention of cancer: misconceptions, *FASEB Journal* 11: 1041–52.
Bowman, W.C. and Rand, M.J., 1980, *Textbook of Pharmacology* 2nd edn, Oxford: Blackwell Scientific.
Carson, R., 1962, *Silent Spring*, New York; Houghton Mifflin.
Frieberg, E.C., Walker, G.C. and Siede, W., 1995, *DNA Repair and Mutagenesis*, Washington DC: ASM Press.
Halliwell, B. and Aruoma, O.I., 1993, *DNA and Free Radicals*, New York: Ellis Harwood.
Kelly, F.J., 1996, Air pollution: an old problem in a new guise, *Biologist* 43: 102–5.
Lear, L., 1997, *Rachel Carson: The Life of the Author of Silent Spring*, Harmondsworth:

Penguin.

Mellanby, K., 1967, *Pesticides and Pollution*, London: Collins.

Wellburn, A., 1994, *Air Pollution and Climate Change: The Biological Impact*, Harlow: Longman Scientific and Technical.

Wingard, L.B., Brody, T.M., Larner, J. and Schwartz, A., 1991, *Human Pharmacology: Molecular to Clinical*, London: Wolfe.

## Chapter 6

Ames, B.N. and Gold, L.S.,1997, Environmental pollution, pesticides and the prevention of cancer: misconceptions, *FASEB Journal* 11: 1041–52.

Aruoma, O.I. and Halliwell B., 1991, *Free Radicals and Food Additives*, London: Taylor & Francis.

Bennion, M., 1980, *The Science of Food*, New York: John Wiley.

Frieberg, E.C., Walker, G.C. and Siede, W., 1995, *DNA Repair and Mutagenesis*, Washington DC: ASM Press.

Halliwell, B. and Aruoma, O.I., 1993, *DNA and Free Radicals*, New York: Ellis Harwood.

Harborne, J.B., 1977, *Introduction to Ecological Biochemistry*, London: Academic Press.

Nottingham, S, 1998, *Eat Your Genes: How Genetically Modified Food is Entering our Diet*, London: Zed Books.

Waldron, K.W., Johnson, I.T. and Fenwick, G.R., 1993, *Food and Cancer Prevention: Chemical and Biological Effects*, London: Royal Society of Chemistry.

Williams, W.R., 1908, *The Natural History of Cancer*, New York: William Wood.

## Chapter 7

Beckman, K.D. and Ames, B.N., 1997, Oxidative decay of DNA, *Journal of Biological Chemistry* 272: 19633–6.

Cann, A.J., 1993, *Principles of Molecular Virology*, London: Academic Press.

Forman, H.J. and Cadenas, E., 1997, *Oxidative Stress and Signal Transduction*, New York: Chapman & Hall.

Frieberg, E.C., Walker, G.C. and Siede, W., 1995, *DNA Repair and Mutagenesis*, Washington DC: ASM Press.

Hahn, S.M., Mitchell, J.B. and Shacter, E., 1997, Tempol inhibits neutrophil and hydrogen peroxide-mediated DNA damage, *Free Radical Biology and Medicine* 23: 879–84.

Halliwell, B. and Aruoma, O.I., 1993, *DNA and Free Radicals*, New York: Ellis Harwood.

Henle, E.S. and Linn, S., 1997, Formation, prevention and repair of DNA damage by iron/hydrogen peroxide, *Journal of Biological Chemistry* 272: 19095–8.

Kwong, L.K. and Sohal, R.S., 1998, Substrate and site specificity of hydrogen peroxide generation in mouse mitochondria, *Archives of Biochemistry and Biophysics* 350: 118–26.

Lindahl, T., 1993, Instability and decay of the primary structure of DNA, *Nature* 362: 706–15.

Rice-Evans, C. and Burdon, R., 1993, Free radical–lipid interactions and their pathological consequences, *Progress in Lipid Research* 32: 71–110.

Scandalios, J.G., 1997, *Oxidative Stress and the Molecular Biology of Antioxidant Responses*, Cold Spring Harbor, NY: Cold Spring Harbor Laboratory Press.

Shacter, E., Beecham, E.J., Covey, J.M., Kohn, K.W. and Potter, M., 1988, Activated neutrophils induced prolonged DNA damage in neighbouring cells, *Carcinogenesis* 9: 2297–304.

Sohal, R.S., 1997, Mitochondria generate superoxide anion radicals and hydrogen peroxide, *FASEB Journal* 11: 1269–70.

Zastawny, T.H., Dabrowska, M., Jaskolski. T., Klimarczyk, M., Kulinski, L., Koszela, A., Szczesniewicz, M., Sliwinska, M., Witkowski, P. and Olinski, R., 1998, Comparison of oxidative base damage in mitochondrial and nuclear DNA, *Free Radical Biology and Medicine* 24: 722–5.

## Chapter 8

Beissart, S. and Granstein, R.D., 1995, UV-induced cutaneous photobiology, *Critical Reviews in Biochemistry and Molecular Biology* 31: 381–404.

Brash, D.E., 1997, Sunlight and the onset of skin cancer, *Trends in Genetics* 13: 410–14.

Cadet, J., Berger, M., Douki, T., Morin, B., Raoul, S., Ravanat, J.-.L and Spinelli, S., 1997, Effects of UV and visible radiation on DNA: final base damage, *Biological Chemistry* 378: 1275–86.

Christie, M., 2000, *The Ozone Layer*, Cambridge: Cambridge University Press.

Frieberg, E.C., Walker, G.C. and Siede, W., 1995, *DNA Repair and Mutagenesis*, Washington DC: ASM Press.

Halliwell, B. and Aruoma, O.I., 1993, *DNA and Free Radicals*, New York: Ellis Harwood.

Kamb, A., 1994, Sun protection factor p53, *Nature* 372: 730–31.

Leffell, D.J. and Brash, D.E., 1996, Sunlight and skin cancer, *Scientific American* 275, July: 38–43.

Lee, J. and Hawtin, N., 1998, Our health in flux, *New Scientist*, 12 December, Inside Science, No. 116.

Mitchell, A., 1999, Burnt offerings, *New Scientist*, 31 July: 26–7.

Stolarski, R., 1997, A bad winter for Arctic ozone, *Nature* 389: 788–9.

Thiele, J.J., Podda, M. and Packer, L., 1997, Tropospheric ozone: an emerging environmental stress to skin, *Biological Chemistry* 378: 1299–305.

Walker, G., 2000, The hole story, *New Scientist*, 25 March: 24–8.

## Chapter 9

Chin, K.-V., Pastan, I. and Gottesman, M.M., 1993, Function and regulation of the human multidrug resistance gene, *Advances in Cancer Research* 60: 157–80.

Croteau, D.K. and Bohr, V.A., 1997, Repair of oxidative damage to nuclear and mitochondrial DNA in mammalian cells, *Journal of Biological Chemistry* 272: 25409–12.

Coon, M.J., Ding, X., Pernecky, S.J. and Vaz, A.D.N., 1992, Cytochrome P450: progress and predictions, *FASEB Journal* 6: 669–73.

Daniel, V., 1993, Glutathione S-transferases: gene structure and regulation of expression, *Critical Reviews in Biochemistry and Molecular Biology* 28: 173–207.

Davies, K.J.A., 1991, *Oxidative Damage and DNA Repair: Chemical, Biological and Medical Aspects*, Oxford: Pergamon Press.

Forman, H.J. and Cadenas, E., 1997, *Oxidative Stress and Signal Transduction*, New York: Chapman & Hall.

Fridovich, I., 1997, Superoxide anion radical ($O_2^-$), superoxide dismutases and related matters, *Journal of Biological Chemistry* 272: 18515–17.

Frieberg, E.C., Walker, G.C. and Siede, W., 1995, *DNA Repair and Mutagenesis*, Washington DC: ASM Press.

Gonzalez, F.J. and Nebert, D.W., 1990, Evolution of the P450 superfamily: animal–plant warfare, molecular drive and human genetic differences in drug oxidation, *Trends in Genetics* 6: 182–86.

Halliwell, B. and Aruoma, O.I., 1993, *DNA and Free Radicals*, New York: Ellis Harwood.

Henle, E.S. and Linn, S., 1997, Formation, prevention and repair of DNA damage by iron/hydrogen peroxide, *Journal of Biological Chemistry* 272: 19095–8.

Jackson, S.P., 1996, The recognition of DNA damage, *Current Opinion in Genetics and Development* 6: 19–25.

Kolodner, R.D., 1995, Mismatch repair: mechanisms and relationship with cancer susceptibility, *Trends in Biochemical Sciences* 237: 397–401.

Leanderson, P., Faresjo, A.O. and Tagesson, C., 1997, Green tea polyphenols inhibit oxidant-induced DNA strand breakage in cultured lung cells, *Free Radical Biology and Medicine* 23: 235–42.

Lewis, D., 1997, Sex, drugs and P450, *Chemistry and Industry*, 20 October: 831–34.

Liang, F., Han, M., Romanieko, P.J. and Jasin, M., 1998, Homology-directed repair is a major double-strand break repair pathway in mammalian cells, *Proceedings of the National Academy of Sciences USA* 95: 5172–77.

Lindahl, R., 1992, Aldehyde dehydrogenases and their role in carcinogenesis, *Critical Reviews in Biochemistry and Molecular Biology* 27: 283–335.

McCance, R.A. and Widdowson, E.M., 1992, *The Composition of Foods*, London: MAFF.

Modrich, P., 1997, Strand-specific mismatch repair in mammalian cells, *Journal of Biological Chemistry* 272: 24727–30.

Metcalf, F., 1986, *The Penguin Dictionary of Modern Humorous Quotations*, London: Penguin.

Morel, F., Shultz, W.A. and Sies, H., 1994, Gene structure and regulation of expression of human glutathione S-transferase alpha, *Biological Chemistry Hoppe-Seyler* 375: 641–49.

Naegli, H., 1995, Mechanisms of DNA damage recognition in mammalian nucleotide excision repair, *FASEB Journal* 9: 1043–50.

Rice-Evans, C. and Miller, N.J., 1995, Antioxidants: the case for fruit and vegetables in the diet, *British Food Journal* 97: 35–40.

Rice-Evans, C., Miller, N., Bolwell, G.P., Bramley, P.M. and Pridham, J.B., 1995, The relative antioxidant activities of plant-derived polyphenoloic flavonoids, *Free Radical Research* 22: 375–83.

Rice-Evans, C.A., Miller, N.J. and Paganga, G., 1996, Structure–antioxidant activity relationships of flavonoids and phenolic acids, *Free Radical Biology and Medicine* 20: 933–56.

Scandalios, J.G., 1992, *Molecular Biology of Free Radical Scavenging Systems*, Cold Spring Harbor, NY: Cold Spring Harbor Laboratory Press.

Scandalios, J.G., 1997, *Oxidative Stress and the Molecular Biology of Antioxidant Responses*, Cold Spring Harbor, NY: Cold Spring Harbor Laboratory Press.

Seeberg, E., Eide, L. and Bjoras, M., 1995, The base excision pathway, *Trends in Biochemical Sciences* 237: 391–7.

Silverman, J.A. and Schrenk, D., 1997, Expression of the multidrug resistance gene in the liver, *FASEB Journal* 11: 308–13.

Waldron,K.W., Johnson, I.T. and Fenwick, G.R., 1993, *Food and Cancer Prevention: Chemical and Biological Effects*, London: Royal Society of Chemistry.

Weaver, D.T., 1995, What to do at an end: DNA double-strand break repair, *Trends in Genetics* 11: 388–92.

Wingard, L.B., Brody, T.M., Larner, J. and Schwartz, A., 1991, *Human Pharmacology, Molecular to Clinical*, London, Wolfe.

Wood, R.D., 1996, DNA repair in eukaryotes, *Annual Review of Biochemistry* 65: 135–67.

## Chapter 10

Alberts, B., Johnson, A., Lewis, J., Raff, M., Roberts, K. and Walter, P., 2002, *Molecular Biology of the Cell*, 4th edn, New York: Garland.

Agarwal, M.L., Taylor, W.R., Chernov, M.V., Chernova, O.B. and Stark, G.R., 1998, The p53 network, *Journal of Biological Chemistry* 273: 1–4.

Ames, B.N., Gold, L.S. and Willett, W.C., 1995, The causes and prevention of cancer, *Proceedings of the National Academy of Sciences, USA* 92: 52258–65.

Ames, B.N., Shigenaga, M.K. and Hagen, T.M., 1993, Oxidants, antioxidants and the degenerative diseases of aging, *Proceedings of the National Academy of Sciences, USA* 90: 7915–22.

Bridges, B.A., 1997, Hypermutation under stress, *Nature* 387: 557–8.

Cai, J. and Jones, D.P. 1998, Superoxide and apoptosis: mitochondrial generation triggered by cytochrome C loss, *Jounal of Biological Chemistry* 237: 11401–14.

Cavenee, W.K. and White, R.L., 1995, The genetic basis of cancer, *Scientific American* 272, March: 50–57.

Cutler, R.G., 1991, Antioxidants and aging, *American Journal of Clinical Nutrition* 53: 373S-9S.

Darby, S.C. and Roman, E., 1996, Links with childhood leukaemia, *Nature* 382: 303–4.

Duke, R.C., Ojcius, D.M. and Young, J.D.-E., 1996, Cell suicide in health and disease, *Scientific American*, December: 48–55.

Gilchrest, B.A. and Bohr, V.A., 1997, Aging processes, DNA damage and repair, *FASEB Journal* 11: 322–30.

Grollman, A.P. and Moriya, M., 1993, Mutagenesis by 8-oxoguanine: the enemy within, *Trends in Genetics* 9: 246–9.

Halliwell, B. and Aruoma, O.I., 1993, *DNA and Free Radicals*, New York: Ellis Harwood.

Harman, D., 1971, Free radical theory of aging: effect of the amount and degree of unsaturation of dietary fat on mortality rate, *Journal of Gerontology* 26: 451–457.

Hollstein, D., Sideransky, D., Vogelstein, B. and Harris, C.C., 1991, p53 mutations in human cancers, *Science* 253: 49–53.

Hsu, I.C., Metcalf, R.A., Sun, T., Welsh, J.A., Wang, N.J. and Harris, C.C., 1991, Mutational hotspot in the p53 gene in human hepatocellular carcinomas, *Nature* 350: 427–28.

Jazwinski, S.M., 1996, Longevity, genes and ageing, *Science* 273: 54–8.

Korsmeyer, S.J., 1995, Regulators of cell death, *Trends in Genetics* 11: 101–105.

Kanugo, M.S., 1994, *Genes and Aging*, Cambridge: Cambridge University Press.

Kerr, J.F.R., Wyllie, A.H. and Currie, A.R., 1972, Apoptosis: a basic biological phenomenon with wide-ranging implications, *British Journal of Cancer* 26: 239–57.

King, R.J.B., 1996, *Cancer Biology*, Harlow: Addison Wesley Longman.

Kirkwood, T., 1999, *Time of Our Lives: Why Ageing is Neither Inevitable Nor Necessary*, London: Weidenfeld & Nicolson.

Leffell, D.J. and Brash, D.E., 1996, Sunlight and skin cancer, *Scientific American* 275, July: 38–43.

Lodish, H., Berk, A., Zipursky, S.L., Matsudaira, P., Baltimore, D. and Darnell, J., 2000, *Molecular Cell Biology*, 4th edn, New York: W.H. Freeman.

Lombard, D.B. and Guarente, L., 1996, Cloning the gene for Werner's syndrome: a diseases with many symptoms of premature aging, *Trends in Genetics* 12: 283–6.

Phillips, D.H. and Venitt, S., *Environmental Mutagenesis*, Oxford: Bios Scientific.

Potten, C.S., 1987, *Perspectives in Mammalian Cell Death*, Oxford: Oxford University Press.

Rosenberg, S.A. and Barry, J.M., 1992, *The Transformed Cell: Unlocking the Mysteries of Cancer*, London: Chapman.

Ruddon, R.W., 1987, *Cancer Biology*, New York; Oxford University Press.

Orr, W.C. and Sohal, R.S., 1994, Extension of life span by overexpression of superoxide dismutase and catalase in *Drosophila melanogaster*, *Science* 263: 1128–30.

Shigenaga, M.K., Hagen, T.M. and Ames, B.N., 1994, Oxidative damage and mitochondrial decay in aging, *Proceeding of the National Academy of Sciences USA* 91: 10771–8.

Sohal, R.S. and Weindriuch, R., 1996, Oxidative stress, caloric restriction and aging, *Science* 273: 59–63.

Trichopoulos, D., Li, F.P. and Hunter, D.L., 1996, What causes cancer?, *Scientific American* 275, September: 50–57.

Waldron, K.W., Johnson, I.T. and Fenwick, G.R., 1993, *Food and Cancer: Chemical and Biological Aspaects*, Cambridge, Royal Society of Chemistry.

Wallace, D.C., 1997, Mitochondrial DNA in aging and disease, *Scientific American* 277: 22–9.

Wiseman, H. and Halliwell, B., 1996, Damage to DNA by reactive oxygen and nitrogen species: role in imflammatory diseases and progression to cancer, *Biochemical Journal* 313: 17–29.

## Chapter 11

Alberts, B., Johnson, A., Lewis, J., Raff, M., Roberts, K. and Walter, P., 2002, *Molecular Biology of the Cell*, 4th edn, New York: Garland.

Brzozowsli, A.M., Pike, A.C.W., Dauter, Z., Hubbard, R.E., Bonn, T., Engstrom, O., Ohman, L., Greene, G.L., Gustafsson, J.-.A. and Carlquist, M., 1997, Molecular basis of agonism and antagonism in the oestrogen receptor, *Nature* 389: 753–8.

Bunyard, P., 1999, It couldn't happen here, *The Ecologist* 29: 402–7.

Bunyard, P. and Poche, P., 1999, Nuclear power: time to end the experiment, *The Ecologist* 29: 386–9.

Busby, C., 1999, Poisoning in the name of progress, *The Ecologist* 29: 395–401.

Edwards, R., 1997, Radiation roulette, *New Scientist*, 11 October: 37–40.

Cadbury, D., 1997, *The Feminization of Nature: Our Future at Risk*, London: Penguin.

Cairns, J., 1978, *Cancer, Science and Society*, San Francisco: W.H. Freeman.

Cariello, N.F. and Skopek, T.R., 1993, *In vivo* mutation at the human HPRT locus, *Trends in Genetics* 9: 322–6.

Coller, H.A. and Thilly, W.G., 1994, Development and applications of mutational spectra technology, *Environmental Science and Technology* 28: 478A-487A.

Frieberg, E.C., Walker, G.C. and Siede, W., 1995, *DNA Repair and Mutagenesis*, Washington DC: ASM Press.

Halliwell, B. and Aruoma, O.I., 1993, *DNA and Free Radicals*, New York: Ellis Harwood.

Harris, R. and Paxman, J., 1982, *A Higher Form of Killing: The Secret Story of Gas and Germ Warfare*, London: Chatto & Windus.

Henry, M., 1999, The woman who knew too much, *The Ecologist* 29: 404–5.

Lodish, H., Berk, A., Zipursky, S.L., Matsudaira, P., Baltimore, D. and Darnell, J., 2000, *Molecular Cell Biology*, 4th edn, New York: W.H. Freeman.

McBride, T.J., Preston, B.D. and Loeb, L.A., 1991, Mutagenic spectrum resulting from DNA damage by oxygen radicals, *Biochemistry* 30: 207–13.

Neel, J.V., 1998, Genetic studies at the Atomic Bomb Casualty Commission–Radiation Effects Research Foundation: 1946–97, *Proceedings of the National Academy of Sciences USA* 95: 5432–36.

Patlak, M., 1997, Fingering carcinogens with genetic evidence, *Environmental Science and Technology* 31: 190A-192A.

Perera, F.P., 1996, Uncovering new clues to cancer risk, *Scientific American* 274, May: 40–6.

Pfeifer, G.P., 1996, *Technologies for Detection of DNA Damage and Mutation*, New York, Plenum Press.

Phillips, D.H. and Venitt, S., 1995, *Environmental Mutagenesis*, Oxford: Bios Scientific.

Rice-Evans, C.A, Halliwell, B. and Lunt, G.G.,1995, *Free Radicals and Oxidative Stress: Environment, Drugs and Food Additives*, London: Portland Press.

Schull, W.J., 1998, The somatic effects of exposure to atomic radiation: the Japanese experience, 1947–1997, *Proceedings of the National Academy of Sciences USA* 95: 5437–41.

Sneader, W., 1985, *Drug Discovery: The Evolution of Modern Medicines*, Chichester: John Wiley.

Steingraber, S., 1998, *Living Downstream: An Ecologist Looks at Cancer and the Environment*, London: Virago.

Thomas, J.A., 1997, Phytoestrogens and hormonal modulation: a mini-review, *Environmental and Nutritional Interactions* 1: 5–12.

Tolonen, M., 1990, *Vitamins and Minerals in Health and Nutrition*, Chichester: Ellis Harwood.

Waldron, K.W., Johnston, I.T. and Fenwick, G.R., 1993, *Food and Cancer Prevention: Chemical and Biological Effects*, London: Royal Society of Chemistry.

Wiman, K.G., 1997, p53: emergency brake and target for cancer therapy, *Experimental Cell Research* 237: 14–18.

Yu, B.P., 1996, Aging and oxidative stress: modulation by dietary restriction, *Free Radical Biology and Medicine* 21: 651–68.

## Chapter 12

Dawkins, R., 1986, *The Blind Watchmaker*, Harlow: Longman Scientific and Technical.
Dawkins, R., 1995, *River Out of Eden*, London: Weidenfeld & Nicolson.
Desmond, A. and Moore, J., 1991, *Darwin*, London: Michael Joseph.
Jones, S., 1999, *Almost Like a Whale: The Origin of Species Updated*, London: Transworld.
Leakey, R.E., 1979, *The Illustrated Origin of Species by Charles Darwin*, London: Faber & Faber.
Lewin, R., 1997, *Patterns in Evolution*, New York: Scientific American Library.
Lewontin, R., 1995, *Human Diversity*, New York: Scientific American Library.
Lewis, C., 2000, *The Dating Game*, Cambridge: Cambridge University Press.
Moorhead, A., 1971, *Darwin and the Beagle*, Harmondsworth: Penguin.
Raup, D.M., 1991, *Extinction: Bad Genes or Bad Luck*, New York: W.W. Norton.

## Chapter 13

An, W.G., Kanekal, M., Simon, M.C., Maltepe, E., Blagosklonny, M.K. and Neckers, L.M., 1998, Stabilization of wild-type p53 by hypoxia-inducible factor $1\alpha$, *Nature*, 329, 405–8.
Burdon, R.H., 1993, Heat shock proteins in relation to medicine, *Molecular Aspects of Medicine* 14: 83–165.
Burdon, R.H., 1993, Stress proteins in plants, *Botanical Journal of Scotland*, 46, 463–75.
Chang, C.-Y. and Puga, A., 1998, Constitutive activation of the aromatic hydrocarbon receptor, *Molecular and Cellular Biology* 18: 525–35.
Chin, K.-V., Pastan, I. and Gottesman, M.M., 1993, Function and regulation of the human multidrug resistance gene, *Advances in Cancer Research* 60: 157–80.
Coon, M.J., Ding, X., Pernecky, S.J. and Vaz, A.D.N., 1992, Cytochrome P450: progress and predictions, *FASEB Journal* 6: 669–73.
Crawford, R.M.M., 1989, *Studies in Plant Survival: Ecological Case Histories of Plant Adaptation to Adversity*, Oxford, Blackwell Scientific.
Crawford, R.M.M., 1993, Plant survival without oxygen, *Biologist* 40: 110–14.
Daniel, V., 1993, Glutathione S-transferases: gene structure and regulation of expression, *Critical Reviews in Biochemistry and Molecular Biology* 28: 173–207.
Drew, M.C., 1997, Oxygen deficiency and root metabolism: injury and acclimation under hypoxia and anoxia, *Annual review of Plant Physiology and Plant Molecular Biology* 48: 223–50.
Fiege, U., Morimoto, R.I., Yahara, I. and Polla, B.S., 1996, *Stress-Inducible Cellular Responses*, Basel: Birkhauser Verlag.
Frohnmeyer, H., Bowler, C. and Schafer, E., 1997, Evidence for some signal

transduction elements involved in UV-light-dependent responses in parsley protoplasts, *Journal of Experimental Botany* 48: 739–50.

Fischer, E.H. and Davie, E.W., 1998, Recent excitement regarding metallothionein, *Proceedings of the National Academy of Sciences USA* 95: 3333–4.

Goldberg, M.A., Dunning, S.P. and Bunn, H.F., 1988, Regulation of the erythropoetin gene: evidence that the oxygen sensor is a haem protein, *Science* 242: 1412–15.

Gonzalez, F.J. and Nebert, D.W., 1990, Evolution of the P450 gene superfamily, *Trends in Genetics* 6: 182–6.

Guy, C.L., 1990, Cold acclimation and freezing stress tolerance: role of protein metabolism, *Annual Review of Plant Physiology and Plant Molecular Biology* 41: 187–223.

Hartl, F.U., 1996, Molecular chaperones in cellular protein folding, *Nature* 381: 571–80.

Harwood, J., 1991, Strategies for coping with low environmental temperatures, *Trends in Biochemical Sciences* 16: 126–7.

Hughes, M.A. and Dunn, M.A.,1996, The molecular biology of plant acclimation to low temperature, *Journal of Experimental Botany* 47: 291–305.

Ingram, J. and Bartels, D., 1996, The molecular basis of dehydration tolerance in plants, *Annual Review of Plant Physiology and Plant Molecular Biology* 47: 377–403.

Jia, Z., DeLuca, C.I., Chao, and Davies, P.L.,1996, Structural basis for the binding of a globular antifreeze protein to ice, *Nature* 384: 285–8.

Madigan, M.T. and Marrs, B.L., 1997, Extremophiles, *Scientific American*, April: 66–71.

McCue, K.F. and Hanson, A.D., 1990, Drought and salt tolerance: towards understanding and application, *Trends in Biotechnology* 8: 358–62.

Mergeay, M., 1991, Towards an understanding of the genetics of bacterial metal resistance, *Trends in Biotechnology* 9: 17–24.

Morimoto, R.I., Tissieres, A. and Georgopoulos, C., 1990, *Stress Proteins in Biology and Medicine*, Cold Spring Harbor, NY: Cold Spring Harbor Laboratory Press.

Morimoto, R. I., Tissieres, A. and Georgopoulos, C., 1994, *The Biology of Heat Shock Proteins and Molecular Chaperones*, Cold Spring Harbor, NY: Cold Spring Harbor Laboratory Press.

Murata, N. and Los, D.A., 1997, Membrane fluidity and temperature perception, *Plant Physiology* 115: 875–879.

Nihida, I. and Murata, N., 1996, Chilling sensitivity in plants and cyanobacteria; the crucial contribution of membrane lipids, *Annual Review of Plant Physiology and Plant Molecular Biology* 47: 541–68.

Prestera, T. and Talalay, P., 1995, Electrophile and antioxidant regulation of enzymes that detoxify carcinogens, *Proceedings of the National Academy of Sciences USA* 92: 8965–9.

Prochaska, H.J. and Talalay, P., 1988, Regulatory mechanisms of monofunctional and bifunctional anticarcinogenic enzyme inducers in murine liver, *Cancer Research* 48: 4776–82.

Ryter, S.W. and Tyrell, R.M., 1998, Singlet molecular oxygen ($^1O_2$): a possible effector of eukaryotic gene expression, *Free Radical Biology and Medicine*, 24, 1520–34.

Scandalios, J.G., 1997, *Oxidative Stress and the Molecular Biology of Antioxidant Responses*, Cold Spring Harbor, NY: Cold Spring Harbor Laboratory Press.

Scandalios, J.G., 1990, *Genomic Responses to Environmental Stress*, London: Academic Press.

Schlesinger, M.J., Ashburner, M. and Tissieres, A., 1982, *Heat Shock: From Bacteria to Man*, Cold Spring Harbor, NY: Cold Spring Harbor Laboratory.

Schlesinger, M.J., Santoro, M.G. and Garaci, E., 1990, *Stress Proteins*, Berlin: Springer Verlag.

Shinozaki, K. and Yamaguchi-Shinozaki, K., 1997, Gene expression and signal transduction in water-stress response, *Plant Physiology* 115: 327–34.

Shmidt-Nielsen, K.,1983, *Animal Physiology: Adaptation and Enviroment*, 3rd edn, Cambridge, Cambridge University Press.

Silverman, J.A. and Schrenk, D., 1997, Expression of the multidrug resistance genes in the liver, *FASEB Journal* 11: 308–13.

Stoop, J., Williamson, J.D. and Mason Pharr, D., 1996, Mannitol metabolism in plants: a method of coping with stress, *Trends in Plant Science* 1: 139–44.

Summers, A.O., 1985, Bacterial resistance to toxic elements, *Trends in Biotechnology* 3: 122–5.

Thiele, D., 1992, Metal-regulated transcription in eukaryotes, *Nucleic Acids Research* 20: 1183–91.

Thomashow, M.F., 1998, Role of cold-responsive genes in plant freezing tolerance, *Plant Physiology*, 118, 1–8.

Wang, G.L. and Semenza, G.L., 1993, Characterization of hypoxia-inducible factor 1 and regulation of DNA binding by hypoxia, *Journal of Biological Chemistry* 268: 21513–18.

Welch, W.J., 1993, How cells respond to stress, *Scientific American*, May: 34–41.

Wellburn, A., 1994, *Air Pollution and Climate Change: The Biological Impact*, Harlow: Longman Scientific and Technical.

Wu, L. and Whitlock Jr., J.P., 1993, Mechanism of dioxin action: receptor-enhancer interactions in intact cells, *Nucleic Acids Research* 21: 119–25.

Yeo, A., 1998, Molecular biology of salt tolerance in the context of whole plant physiology, *Journal of Experimental Botany* 49: 915–24.

## Chapter 14

Alberts, B., Johnson, A., Lewis, J., Raff, M., Roberts, K. and Walter, P., 2002, *Molecular Biology of the Cell*, 4th edn, New York: Garland.

Adams, R.L.P. and Burdon, R.H., 1985, *The Molecular Biology of DNA Methylation*,

New York, Spriger Verlag.

Bellamy, D. and Quayle, B., 1986, *Turning the Tide*, London: William Collins.

Daniell, H., Datta, R., Varma, S., Gray, S. and Lee, S.-B., 1998, Containment of herbicide resistance through genetic engineering of the chloroplast genome, *Nature Biotechnology* 16: 345–48.

De la Fuente, J.M., Ramirez-Rodriguez, V., Cabrera-Ponce, J.L. and Herrera-Estrella, L., 1997, Aluminium tolerance in transgenic plants by alteration of citrate synthesis, *Science* 276: 1566–8.

Dickinson, C.H. and Lucas, J.A., 1982, *Plant Pathology and Plant Pathogens*, 2nd edn, Oxford: Blackwell Scientific.

Fitter, A.H. and Hay, R.K.M., 1987, *Environmental Physiology of Plants*, London: Academic Press.

Gosden, R, 1999, *Designer Babies: The Brave New World of Reproductive Technology*, London: Phoenix.

Jones, P.A., 1996, DNA Methylation Errors and Cancer, *Cancer Research* 56: 2463–7.

Kolata, G., 1997, *Clone: The Road to Dolly and the Path Ahead*, Harmondsworth: Penguin.

Lodish, H., Berk, A., Zipursky, S.L., Matsudaira, P., Baltimore, D. and Darnell, J., 2000, *Molecular Cell Biology*, 4th edn, New York: W.H. Freeman.

Murata, N., Ishizaki-Nishizawa, O., Higashi, S., Hayashi, H., Tasaka, Y. and Nishida, I., 1992, Genetically engineered alteration in the chilling sensitivity of plants, *Nature* 356: 710–13.

Nottingham, S., 1998, *Eat Your Genes: How Genetically Modified Food is Entering our Diet*, London: Zed Books.

Nottingham, S., 2002, *Genescapes: The Ecology of Genetic Engineering*, London: Zed Books.

Rogers, H.J. and Parkes, H.C., 1995, Transgenic plants and the environment, *Journal of Experimental Botany* 46: 467–88.

Song, W.-Y., Wang, G.-L., Chen, L.-L., Kim, H.-S., Pi, L.-Y., Holste, T., Gardner, J., Wang, B., Zhai, W.-X., Zhu, L.-H., Faquet, C. and Ronald, P. 1995, A receptor kinase-like protein encoded by the rice disease resistance gene, *Xa21*, *Science* 270: 1804–06.

## Chapter 15

Ames, B.N. and Gold, L.S., 1997, Environmental pollution, pesticides, and the prevention of cancer: misconceptions, *FASEB Journal* 11: 1041–52.

Bell, Peter and Woodcock, Christopher, 1971, *The Diversity of Green Plants*, 2nd edn, London: Edward Arnold.

Brodribb, J., 1997, Mission earth, *New Scientist*, 13 December, Inside Science, No. 106.

Bunyard, P., 1999, It couldn't happen here, *The Ecologist* 29: 402–7.

Bunyard, P. and Poche, P., 1999, Nuclear power: time to end the experiment, *The Ecologist* 29: 386–9.

Busby, C., 1999, Poisoning in the name of progress, *The Ecologist* 29: 395–401.

Edwards, R., 1997, Radiation roulette, *New Scientist*, 11 October: 37–40.

Cadbury, D., 1997, *The Feminization of Nature*, Harmondsworth, Penguin.

Dobson, A.P., 1996, *Conservation and Biodiversity*, New York: Scientific American Library, W.H. Freeman.

Epstein, S., 1998, Winning the war against cancer?… Are they even fighting it? *The Ecologist* 28: 69–80.

Fraser, P.J. and Prather, M.J., 1999, Uncertain road to ozone recovery, *Nature* 398: 663–4.

Glazer, A.N. and Nikaido, H., 1995, *Microbial Biotechnology*, New York: W.H. Freeman.

Goldsmith, Z., 1998, Cancer: a disease of industrialization, *The Ecologist* 28: 93–9.

Leakey, R. and Lewin, R., 1996, *The Sixth Extinction: Biodiversity and its Survival*, London: Weidenfeld & Nicolson.

Lodovic, M., 1994, Effect of a mixture of 15 commonly used pesticides on DNA levels of 8-hydroxy-2-deoxyguanosine and xenobiotic metabolizing enzymes in rat liver, *Journal of Environmental Pathology, Toxicology and Oncology* 13: 163–8.

Maloy, S.R., Cronan, J.E. and Freifelder, D., 1994, *Microbial Genetics*, 2nd edn, Boston, MA: Jones & Bartlett.

McEldowney, S., Hardman, D.J. and Waite, S., 1993, *Pollution: Ecology and Biotreatment*, Harlow: Longman Scientific and Technical.

Phillips, D.H. and Venitt, S., 1995, *Environmental Mutagenesis*, Oxford: Bios Scientific.

Salt, D.E., Smith, R.D. and Raskin, I., 1998, Phytoremediation, *Annual Review of Plant Physiology and Plant Molecular Biology* 49: 643–68.

Scandalios, J., 1990, *Genomic Responses to Environmental Stress*, San Diego: Academic Press.

Scandalios, J., 1997, *Oxidative Stress and the Molecular Biology of Antioxidant Defenses*, Cold Spring Harbor, NY: Cold Spring Harbor Laboratory Press.

Spielman, A. and D'Antonio, 2002, *Mosquito*, London: Faber & Faber.

Steingraber, S., 1998, *Living Downstream: An Ecologist Looks at Cancer and the Environment*, London, Virago Press.

Terborough, John, 1992, *Diversity and the Tropical Rainforest*, New York: Scientific American Library.

Vines, G., 1999, Mass extinctions, *New Scientist, Inside Science*, 126.

Waldron, K.W., Johnson, I.T. and Fenwick, G.R., 1993, *Food and Cancer Protection: Chemical and Biological Aspects*, Cambridge: Royal Society of Chemistry.

Watanabe, M.Y., 1997, Phytoremediation on the brink of commercialization, *Environmental Science and Technology* 31: 1.

Wellburn, A., 1994, *Air Pollution and Climate Change, The Biological Impact*, Harlow:

Addison Wesley Longman.

Wellington, E.M.H. and Van Elsa, J.D., *Genetic Interactions among Microorganisms in the Natural Environment*, Oxford: Pergamon Press.

White, A., 1998, Children, pesticides and cancer, *The Ecologist* 28: 100–105.

## General

Burdon, R.H., 1999, *Genes and the Environment*, London: Taylor & Francis.

Crick, F., 1981, *Life Itself: Its Origin and Nature*, London: Macdonald.

Crick, F., 1990, *What Mad Pursuit: A Personal View of Scientific Discovery*, Harmondsworth: Penguin.

Cunningham, W.P. and Saigo, B.W., 1990, *Environmental Science: A Global Concern*, Dubuque, IA: William C. Brown.

Davies, P., 1999, *The Fifth Miracle: The Search for the Origin of Life*, Harmondsworth: Penguin.

Garrett, L., 1994, *The Coming Plague: Newly Emerging Diseases in a World Out of Balance*, New York; Penguin Books.

Gribbin, J. and Gribbin, M., 1996, The greenhouse effect, *New Scientist*, 6 July, Inside Science, No. 92.

Halliwell, B. and Gutteridge, J.M.C., 1998, *Free Radicals in Biology and Medicine*, 3rd edn, Oxford: Clarendon Press.

Hazen, R.M. and Trefil, J., 1996, *The Physical Sciences: An Integrated Approach*, New York: John Wiley.

Hughes, M.A., 1996, *Plant Molecular Genetics*, Harlow: Addison Wesley–Longman.

Jacob, F., 1998, *Of Flies, Mice and Men*, Cambridge, MA: Harvard University Press.

Karl, T.R., Nicholls, N. and Gregory, J., 1997, The coming climate, *Scientific American*, May, 55–9.

Kaufman, P. B., 1989, *Plants: Their Biology and Importance*, New York: Harper & Row.

Kaufmann, W. J. III, 1997, *Discovering the Universe*, New York: W.H. Freeman.

Lomberg, B., 2001, *The Skeptical Environmentalist: Measuring the Real State of the World*, Cambridge: Cambridge University Press .

Mayr, E., 1997, *This is Biology: The Science of the Living World*, Cambridge, MA: Harvard University Press.

McNeill, J., 2000, *Something New Under the Sun: An Environmental History of the Twentieth Century*, London: Allen Lane.

Pollack, R., 1994, *Signs of Life: The Language and Meanings of DNA*, London: Viking.

Rice-Evans, C.A. and Burdon R.H., 1994, *Free Radical Damage and its Control*, Amsterdam: Elsevier Science.

Ridley, M., 1999, *Genome: The Autobiography of a Species in 23 Chapters*, London: Fourth Estate.

Wilson, E.O., 1992, *The Diversity of Life*, Harmondsworth: Penguin.
Zimmerman, M., 1997, *Science, Nonscience and Nonsense: Approaching Environmental Literacy*, Baltimore, MD: Johns Hopkins University Press.

# Index

## Zed Books Titles on
## Genetic Engineering and Biotechnology

Scientific advances in biology, the ability to engage in genetic engineering, the inclusion of genetic material under the protective umbrella of intellectual property rights and the commercial interests of the handful of giant corporations who dominate research and development in these fields have created a potent cocktail of change. This nexus of power and technical capacities raise extraordinarily important issues relating to the ethics of manipulating nature, the consequences for human health, biodiversity and protection of the environment, and social questions including the implications for Third World farmers and food security in the South. Zed Books is developing a strong list on the social, environmental and ethical dimensions of these questions.

M. Avramovic, *An Affordable Development? Biotechnology, Economics and the Implications for the Third World*

Robert Ali Brac de la Perrière and Franck Seuret, *Brave New Seeds: The Threat of GM Crops to Farmers*

Roy Burdon, *The Suffering Gene: Environmental Threats to Our Health*

Stephen Nottingham, *Eat Your Genes: How Genetically Modified Food is Entering Our Diet*

Stephen Nottingham, *Genescapes: The Ecology of Genetic Engineering*

Helena Paul and Ricarda Steinbrecher, with Lucy Michaels, Devlin Kuyek, *Feeding the Hungry TNCs: Corporate Colonization of the Food Chain*

Vandana Shiva and Caroline Moser (eds), *Biopolitics: Perspectives on Biodiversity and Biotechnology*

Brian Tokar (ed.), *Redesigning Life? The Worldwide Challenge to Genetic Engineering*

For full details of this list and Zed's other subject and general catalogues, please write to: The Marketing Department, Zed Books, 7 Cynthia Street, London N1 9JF, UK or email Sales@zedbooks.demon.co.uk

Visit our website at: www.zedbooks.demon.co.uk